Dancing with Dementia

My Story of Living Positively with Dementia

Christine Bryden

Jessica Kingsley *Publishers*
London and Philadelphia

Cover photograph by Danny O'Neill

First published in 2005
by Jessica Kingsley Publishers
73 Collier Street
London N1 9BE, UK
and
400 Market Street, Suite 400
Philadelphia, PA 19106, USA

www.jkp.com

Library of Congress Cataloging in Publication Data
Bryden, Christine, 1949-
  Dancing with dementia : my story of living positively with dementia / Christine Bryden.
   p. cm.
  Includes bibliographical references.
  ISBN 1-84310-332-X (pbk.)
  1. Bryden, Christine, 1949---Mental health. 2. Dementia--Patients--Biography. 3. Alzhei-
mer's disease--Patients--Biography. I. Title.
  RC523.3.B79 2005
  362.196'831'0092--dc22

                                                    2004021146

British Library Cataloguing in Publication Data
A CIP catalogue record for this book is available from the British Library

ISBN 978 1 84310 332 5
eISBN 978 1 84642 095 5

Printed and bound in Great Britain

To my husband Paul, who is God's precious gift to me, walking alongside me in faith and hope for our future. To my daughters Ianthe, Rhiannon and Micheline, who continue to be my best friends as we travel this roller-coaster of life together.

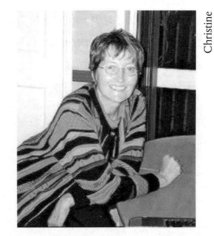

Christine

Contents

PREFACE   9

1   A 'Roller-coaster' Journey Since Early 1998   15
    I'm *really* getting better!!!!   15
    A new lease of life!   23

2   'Coming Out' With Dementia   39
    Challenging the stereotype   39
    Taking the first step   51
    Going global   57
    Whatever next!   74
    Round the world in 80 days   76
    I wouldn't recommend that you move…   85

3   Let's Talk About Having Dementia   89
    The medical journey   89
    What it feels like to live with dementia   97
    There are many ways to help   122

4   I Know Who I'll Be When I Die   155
    An identity crisis!   155
    The fear of ceasing to be   157
    Who am I becoming?   158
    Dancing with dementia   163
    Choosing to dance   166

AFTERWORD   173
APPENDIX 1: DO YOU BELIEVE IN MIRACLES?   175
APPENDIX 2: FREQUENTLY ASKED QUESTIONS   182
APPENDIX 3: WHERE TO GO FOR HELP   197
ENDNOTES   198

Preface

I was sitting, curled up in my favourite chair, with my cat purring contentedly beside me. There was a knock at the door – it was a parcel delivery. As I opened the package, I realised it was two copies of my first book, *Who will I be when I die?*, which was published in 1998.[1] That book talked about my diagnosis with Alzheimer's Disease, a type of dementia, in 1995. At the time of diagnosis I was just 46 years old, in a demanding job in the Prime Minister's Department, and was a single mother with three daughters aged 9 through to 19.

I thought, 'Oh no! That will be the last two copies for me, before they stop publishing the book.' But it was a congratulatory letter from the publisher, sending me two copies of the first reprint. I have had a few more of these letters, and copies of more reprints. And now the book has been translated into Japanese and Chinese, exported to the USA, is to be published in Korea, and has been warmly received by readers in many countries.

When I give talks about what it is like to have dementia and what you can do to help us, people always come up to me and say how much they have enjoyed my first book, how they have lent it to so many other people who have been helped by it to understand more about a loved one with dementia, whether this is Alzheimer's Disease or any of the other forms of dementia. And they always ask when am I going to write another book, so that more people will be able to find out more about what it is like to travel this journey with dementia, and what has happened since the publication of my first book. People with dementia also write to me and say how it had spoken to them, expressed how they felt. My dear Canadian friend wrote 'Thank you, Christine, for giving words to my thoughts, my feelings, my life.'[2]

You see, my life has done an amazing turnaround since 1998, when I was expected to go into a nursing home by 2000 and maybe die by 2004. I have lived another few twists and turns of the roller-coaster of life since then, and have been involved locally, nationally and internationally in the Alzheimer's movement. It is now 2004, and I am still here, and it has been quite a journey of understanding, of seeing more clearly who I am now, who I am becoming, and who I will be when I die.

So what was it that finally tipped the scales in favour of my getting back to my computer to write? It was when Yuji Kawamura, a producer from NHK, the Japanese TV broadcaster in Japan, wrote to me and asked if he could do a TV Special. The letter said:

> A few days ago I read [the] book again and am impressed that you not only coped with the fear of dementia but also found a deeper, or newer 'self' out of your experience. I also read the draft copy of your lecture and realized that your process of trying to know yourself even deepened since you wrote the book. If we could show people how you are living a more profound, fulfilling life than before, I believe society would change, as well as the care of dementia itself.[3]

In my first book I had written about how I got steadily worse, but then seemed to be getting just a little better, over the three years after that devastating diagnosis. I spoke about my spiritual, emotional and physical journey with dementia. And although I felt a lot better towards the end of writing the book, I had no other choice but to turn to my faith. Medically the prospects were hopeless – steady decline into increasing dementia as more and more of my brain shrivelled up and died. My book title – *Who will I be when I die?* – reflected the fear of losing self, of a future without knowledge of identity.

But in my talks now, I reflect on a journey of living positively with dementia, and of discovering a journey into the centre of self. I speak to professional care-givers, families, medical professionals, and others, telling them what we feel like, what we need, and trying to give hope and understanding in the face of this mystery illness that robs us of who we think we are. Whilst advocating urgently for a cure, we need to improve understanding and treatment of those living with dementia.

It has been a long and interesting struggle of advocacy for people with dementia, first to my local, then to national Alzheimer's Associations, from 1998 to 2001. Then I made contact with the international Alzheimer's movement, and an important part of this journey was meeting Noriko Ishibashi in Christchurch in 2001. Somehow we managed to connect at the level of emotion and spirit, across language and culture. She has become a dear friend, and has achieved the publication of my book in Japanese, and has been a great source of encouragement in writing this second book.

By 2003 I had been elected to the Board of Alzheimer's Disease International to represent people with dementia. It is now mid 2004, and I am still struggling and surviving, and doing all I can to change the perceptions we have of dementia. But why have I tried so hard? Why have I been so public about my disease? I don't like all the attention, but the reason I have done all of this is because I hope that one day we will treat these physical diseases of the brain like any other disease of our body.

One day I hope that we will treat people with dementia with respect, recognise just how hard they are trying to cope with getting through each day, and provide them with appropriate emotional support, social networks and encouragement. One day I hope there will be a cure. There are 24 million people around the world who are living with dementia, who are worthy of respect and should be regarded as an international treasure.

Each person with dementia is travelling a journey deep into the core of their spirit, away from the complex cognitive outer layer that once defined them, through the jumble and tangle of emotions created through their life experiences, into the centre of their being, into what truly gives them meaning in life. Many of us seek earnestly for this sense of the present time, the sense of 'now', of how to live each moment and treasure it as if it were the only experience to look at and to wonder at. But this is the experience of dementia, life in the present without a past or future.

Looking back, it has been an amazing journey of self-discovery, change and growth. Working with other friends with dementia around the world, and their supporters, I see changes in the way dementia is viewed, and I hope for a better understanding. By writing this book, as well as my first book, and giving many talks, I have done all that I can to help change attitudes.

But this book has been an enormous struggle to write. It has taken six years, of collecting together various talks that I have given, papers that I have written, and emails that were exchanged between me and my friends with dementia. Even then, it made no sense until I talked about my ideas with others, particularly with Yuji Kawamura and Liz MacKinlay. My husband, Paul, has been my faithful co-worker, encouraging me on those many occasions when it all felt too much, and helping me to remember all the many events over the years, giving me clues, ideas, prompts and recollections. We have shared many laughs at my confusions and funny expressions.

IT IS TIME to rest, and I can add little to those words of Ronald Reagan, when he said 'I plan to enjoy the great outdoors and stay in touch with my friends and supporters… I now begin the journey that will lead me into the sunset of my life.'[4]

I plan to treasure each moment that remains with my family and my friends, hoping that I remain well enough long enough to benefit from any cure that might be discovered. But I know that in the first part of this dance with dementia, I did what I could with the energy I had left to reach out to help others to gain a better understanding of people with dementia and the care that we need in our journey.

For me, my Christian faith is very much part of why and how I try to live positively each day with dementia. I hope that my belief, or your different faith tradition or unbelief, does not cloud the real message of hope in living each day to the full, treasuring each moment as if it were your last.

There are so many people in my life to thank, more than I can possibly name. All I can do is to say is that without the support of my family, of the Alzheimer's movement, and of my Christian friends, I could not cope with this daily struggle. This book would not have become a reality without the encouragement and enthusiasm of Noriko Ishibashi, Yasuji Ishikura, Yuji Kawamura, Eiji Tajima and Yoko Higaki. Revd Dr Liz MacKinlay, my friend and my spiritual advisor, has helped me with reading and editing, reflecting on what I am trying to say, and she is my very dear friend and sister-in-Christ.

I am so grateful to my friends, who also are living with dementia, in the Dementia Advocacy and Support Network International. Without their support and encouragement, and sharing, I would feel very alone. In particular, I want to acknowledge the inspiration and insight that Morris Friedell has given me directly and to all of us in this network. He has been able to express our aspirations, our fears and our search for identity in our struggle with dementia.

My neurologist has walked with me every step of the way, carefully assessing me each year, being realistic yet positive, and giving me hope. I am indebted to him for empowering me to live life to the full despite my diagnosis with dementia.

But most of all I thank Paul, Ianthe, Rhiannon, Micheline and Rachel, who are my best friends as we walk this roller-coaster of life together. We are adjusting our dance steps to the changing melody of dementia, listening to the music within, as well as being encouraged by the supportive music around us.

1

A 'Roller-coaster' Journey Since Early 1998

I'm *really* getting better!!!!

My eldest daughter, Ianthe, and I were sitting in the quiet, window-less waiting room in Sydney, for me to be seen by the neurologist for my yearly check up, to see how I was going with my Alzheimer's Disease, how the medications were affecting me, and whether there were any functional or mood changes that I had noticed in myself.

It was cool inside and there was very little noise, apart from the clack, clack, clack of the receptionists' keypads, and the rustling of magazine pages being idly turned. It was May 1998, and outside Sydney bustled busily in the sunshine of a warm autumn day.

I tried to focus on the article in the nature magazine before me, but inside I was bubbling over with excitement. I wanted to rush in and shout 'I'm better!' – but Ianthe, bless her soul, had been able to restrain me and suggest that perhaps if I did this the neurologist would definitely think I had 'lost it' and was declining further into my dementia.

We had talked about this in the car during the long three-hour drive on the highway from Canberra to Sydney, and she suggested that maybe I should try to stay calm and simply say, 'I think I'm beginning to feel a lot better at the moment'.

Calm?! I felt far from calm. This was hugely exciting, this was the most amazing thing that had ever happened in my life. This was something unheard of – in all of my reading about Alzheimer's I had never ever seen anything about people doing anything other than declining. Sure, they might stabilise for a while, especially on the new anti-dementia drugs. But feel better? No, that never happened.

1995–1998

At first, after my diagnosis in May 1995, for a year or so I really did feel as though nothing was really wrong, and maybe it was all a mistake. But I enjoyed the time off work to be with my daughters and to rest with fewer weekly migraines. And in October 1995, the neurologist started me on Tacrine (Cognex), which was the first breakthrough drug for mild to moderate dementia, just on the Australian market. It was an anti-cholinesterase inhibitor.

These types of drug stop the breakdown of acetyl choline in the brain. So, what's so special about acetyl choline? Well, it's a chemical messenger in the brain making the neurones spark better and speak to each other more clearly. Basically you get better reception inside your head if you have more acetyl choline inside there. With diseases like Alzheimer's and other dementias, acetyl choline tends to be in short supply, so your brain gets very slow and 'foggy-feeling' inside. By taking one of these anti-cholinesterase inhibitors, you get to increase the level of chemical messenger, and so help what remains to function better. It's a bit like a staircase on the sinking ocean liner, the Titanic, taking me to a higher deck, so my feet won't get wet as soon! Not a cure, but what's called a symptomatic treatment.

But even with more of this stuff sloshing around inside my brain, by mid to late 1996, I began to notice real changes, difficulties in functioning, in remembering, in speaking, in all sorts of things. Before I thought it was only a little problem, which could be excused due to stress. And even when faced with the awful picture of damage on the scans, I explained it all away by saying to myself that maybe I had always had this physical brain damage that showed on the scans, but had managed very well with what I had. I felt a bit of a fraud, to tell you the truth!

But by early 1997, there was no question that something was seriously wrong with me, and no amount of extra chemical messenger was going to really mask this. I had really deteriorated, changing as a person, losing the super-fast, super-smart me. I had become much slower in my speech, less able to make decisions, and more readily confused. As I slowed down further, it was as if the world was too fast for me. So much so that by mid 1997, I could not have given any talks, and I struggled to finish my first book. I was well into my journey with the disease, experiencing most of the cognitive, behavioural and neurological signs of mild to moderate dementia. I no longer drove, answered the phone or watched TV, but retreated into gardening and books, as well as very early bedtimes.

I was sinking into depression, believing the medical model of inexorable decline with dementia. And depression leads to pseudo-dementia, where you show more symptoms of dementia than might be expected from your brain damage. I was on a downward spiral of hopelessness and despair, as a result of which I was withdrawing into dysfunction. Alongside this depression were some very real symptoms of the dementia.

I began to experience hallucinations, which I found very scary, and finally asked three people at my church to pray for these to stop. I wrote briefly about this in my first book.[5] It's since writing that book that I have been told what really happened. Because I had closed my eyes dutifully while these three friends were praying, I had no idea that a whole bunch of my congregation had crowded round me – a bit like a rugby scrum – and prayed for me. And of course these wonderful people had no idea I had set limitations on what to pray for – simply that the hallucinations would stop – so they all prayed fervently for my complete healing. Apparently, so I learned a year or so later, there was even someone visiting that day from the UK, who in the past had been gifted in praying for healing. What a coincidence – or should I say 'God-incidence'?

The hallucinations stopped that day, and I have only had a few minor reminders of what they were like since – usually in the late evening, just as I lie down to sleep, and it seems to be if I am very tired or have started new tablets. I was happy enough to be free of hallucinations, but then over the next month or so, my head began to clear of the fuzzy 'cotton-wool' type of feeling that it felt like before. I could concentrate better, and found it easier to speak and listen. Was this the depression lifting, or was it more than that?

I hadn't expected any more from the prayer than stopping the hallucinations, so it took me a while to realise that I was actually feeling better – definitely not something that was meant to be happening to me, nor what I had expected at all.

I began to speak on the phone again, and even to start driving again, despite the reservations of my eldest daughter, who was naturally quite alarmed at the thought of me in charge of a vehicle.[6] I speak of these improvements in my book, which was finished in February 1998.

But what I didn't write about was that no one believed me when I said I was feeling better, and no longer declining as fast. It was hard enough for my three girls to adjust to the idea – and there was no proof, really. Well, not concrete proof anyway. I just seemed to be more of 'my old self' again. Maybe less depressed?

And given that it was my church friends who had prayed for me to get better, you'd think they would have been the first to believe me, but they weren't. Somehow, everyone still treated me with 'kid gloves', assuming I couldn't do things, so not asking me to.

But looking back now, in early 1998 was when my exciting 'roller-coaster' journey really started, when all sorts of things began to happen which I could never have dreamed were possible.

The neurologist's re-assessment in 1998

But let's go back to the neurologist's office, in May 1998, and the beginning of my quest to prove that I really was feeling better, and battling to survive the decline of dementia by making sure I had a positive attitude. I wanted to hold onto my belief in overcoming the medical model, in allowing the unexpected to invade my life, and to allow my faith to carry me through this struggle to survive.

'Christine?' said the neurologist as he came out of his office, picking up my manila folder from the receptionist's desk, looking toward Ianthe and me with a welcoming smile. I stood up, barely able to contain my excitement, walked in, and said, before I even sat down, 'I'm *really* getting better,' in quite a firm voice, grinning widely. It was hardly something to look down in the mouth about or whisper!

'Well, that's good to hear. It seems as if you are really fighting this disease at the moment. Make the most of this temporary honeymoon,' he responded.

The neurologist's words weren't at all what I wanted to hear! Couldn't he *hear* what I was saying. Didn't he *believe* me? This was no mere stabilisation. This was no *temporary honeymoon*! I was feeling better each day. So I launched into a description of what had been happening to me over the last year.

What exactly had been happening? It had been a year of surprises, of trying to adjust to feeling better, and of then taking up this challenge to move on and make the most of the rest of my life. The words that best expressed how I felt were those said to the crippled man by Jesus, as he healed him: 'Take up your mat and walk'. That is what I felt I had done, take up my mat to start walking this journey of life in faith, to believe I was really able to do more than I had done before.

I thought back to my previous appointment the last August. 'No, I really am getting better. I drive locally again, I feel less confused and I finished the book and sent it to the publishers in January. I felt so much better, so much clearer in the head, that in February – just a few months ago – I enrolled to do a degree in Theology.' This is where Ianthe chipped in: 'Mum even got a High Distinction on one of her assignments!'

After talking with me for a little while longer, the neurologist asked me to sit up on his examination couch, and he got out his little hammer so he could check my reflexes. He also scraped my hand with something sharp, whilst peering intently at my face. What on earth did my face have to do with my hand? Ianthe asked what all these tests were. He replied, 'Your Mum had reverted to some primitive reflexes, which we see in newborn babies, and which are typical of the type of brain damage we see on her scans. This one (when he scraped the hand and looked at my face) is the pout palmar reflex, this one (when he scraped the inside of my hand and looked at my fingers curling up) the grasp one.'

'Hmm.' Then he peered into my eyes with a bright light. 'You do seem to be a bit better. Some of these reflexes are not as strong as they were. Would you mind if we did some more tests?' Would I mind? Of course not, I felt better and was sure that any test would prove it!

So off I went for all the tests again: more scans to check on how the brain damage was progressing, and more psychometric tests to test how my brain – my mind – was functioning.

The scans I had straight away, walking around St Vincent's Specialist Centre, finding all the relevant departments with Ianthe's help. The first was the computer-assisted tomography or CT scan, which would show how much of my brain was damaged. The second was the radio nuclide brain perfusion study, which looked at how what remained of my brain was actually functioning.

For this perfusion study, I was asked to lie quietly in a darkened room, with cotton wool in my ears for half an hour, then I was told a technician would come in and insert a needle in my arm, and that I was not to look at or speak to this person, as they wanted my brain to be 'resting'. Then someone would come in and take me to be scanned. It was a shock to be taken out into the corridor, after all this quiet rest, through into the noisy clatter of the brightly lit scanning room. I lay down onto a table, with a wheel-like scanner slowly clacking its way around my head making its own picture of what it saw inside.

Both the CT and the radio nuclide perfusion scans showed much the same picture – lots of damage, much more than you'd expect for a healthy 49-year-old. And this damage was in the middle, and around the front and sides of the brain. What did all this mean?

The neurologist had arranged for me to have psychometric tests in Canberra, after we got back. These tests involve sitting quietly with a clinical psychologist for two to four hours of questions and 'games'. I managed to see the same lady I had seen for my first diagnosis, and she welcomed me with a warm smile. Dark, short, neat hair, pleated skirt and simple blouse, she had a soft, kind voice. I felt very comfortable, not rushed or stressed, nor put under any sort of pressure.

But then the testing started. The psychologist slowly said numbers, long strings of them, and then asked me to repeat them backwards and forwards. How on earth was I supposed to remember these? Somehow only the last number or two she had said were ringing somewhere inside my head, obliterating any pictures or memories of a series of numbers. I repeated as quickly as I could those few numbers that were echoing loudly in my head, then made a guess as to what might have come next.

Then she told me little stories, asking me questions about them. At first she did this immediately, but then she asked me more questions about these stories after I had done other tests, and of course by then I had forgotten the details of where it had all happened, who had done what, and why and when it was!

She carefully spoke aloud a shopping list, but it was very odd, not like any you might write to go to the supermarket. It had furniture, vegetables, meat, clothes, all sorts of things mixed up together. It was impossible to hang onto the names of enough of the items as she spoke them all out, long enough to try to sort them into any category. All I could do was lamely try to recall as many of the objects as possible. There simply was not enough space inside my brain to do any sorting into types of objects, so that it would be easier to recall them later.

To sort, not only did I have to remember the objects, then label them as a category, but then I had to sort them into each category. It did not end there, because then I had to recall each category, and identify and list what I had remembered in each category. You see, that all takes a huge amount of space up, and I was running out of space inside my head rapidly! As she spoke, I could almost feel bits of the list falling out again, so it was impossible to hold onto enough items to sort and recall.

I remember, too, being given puzzle shapes to put together in a pattern. 'Just take your time,' she said. But no amount of time would help me make sense of the shapes. They simply did not seem to make a pattern. 'It's OK,' she said, 'you still have more time.' But time was not what I needed, I needed something or someone to show me what this all meant. To me, these shapes and these story pictures had no connection to each other that I could see.

For most of these tests she used a stop-watch to record my time. I knew I was slow, so felt further demoralised in that it was being recorded for everyone – or at least her and my doctor – to see. 'Tick, tick, tick,' her watch loudly proclaimed, and my brain seemed even slower than the second hand on the stop watch, as I tried to make sense of all the puzzles laid out before me, the stories told to me, the lists of numbers to recall, the items to remember.

Thankfully, she decided *not* to do the maze test with me again, deciding there was little to be gained by showing that my skills (or lack of them) might have further declined from a previously recorded pretty low level. This was back in 1995. I had sat for what seemed a very long time, in front of a grey inanimate maze, and the psychologist asked me to use an electric rod to trace a path from the top to the bottom. This worked fine for what seemed like just a millisecond, until I made a wrong turn. An electronic buzzer sounded, loudly and insistently, feeling as if it had decimated what was left of my brain.

Carefully I traced the rod through another turn in the maze, but somehow my eyes could not 'see' a path through. There was the beginning, I could see that, and down there somewhere out of my vision was the end. But there was just a muddle of blockages, turns and twists in-between. The buzzer sounded many times, as I desperately sought to make my way from one end of the maze to the other. My score was pitifully low, a mere eighth percentile, and just confirmed what I knew – that I had great difficulty finding my way along unfamiliar routes. It was a great relief not to have to repeat this awful experience again in 1998. After around four hours of testing, with numbers, patterns and stories, somehow she managed to gather all this together to make sense of what was wrong with me.

Her reports were sent to my neurologist, as part of his reassessment. She reported further mild decline, and indications of functional problems in the frontal and temporal areas. The neurologist decided to follow up with another scan, in July 1998, one that might be able to distinguish between the functional patterns of the various types of dementia, a positron emission tomography or PET scan. I knew what I was in for – I had already had a PET scan in 1995, and described this ordeal in my book.[7] You lie there with a mask on your face, your whole body laid out on a metal trolley and wheeled into this small tube. You have needles in each arm – one to put stuff in, the other to take stuff out. You have a blindfold on and ear plugs in, so that you are isolated from the world around you, and very quietly people glide in and out to take samples, or whatever, from the needles in your arms. It seems like hours that you are trapped like this, but in reality it's about 45 minutes.

The PET scanner was in Sydney, so I would need to travel back again from Canberra. It uses radioactive isotopes which have a very short half life, so need to be rushed across the road from the cyclotron to be injected into you, as you lie in a tunnel with a scanner noisily clunking around you, in the Royal Prince Alfred Hospital. Not something for the claustrophobic, I can assure you!

Finally I got the call to come to Sydney for the PET scan. But I will get ahead of myself if I tell you who took me to the bus station in Canberra that blustery July morning. Winter had set in, with early morning frosts and fogs over Canberra. But spring was on the horizon in more ways than I could imagine.

A new lease of life!

The sand felt warm and finely grained between my toes and I squinted against the harsh sun in the glaringly blue sky. Shading my eyes with my hand, I could just make out the dive boat out on the coral reef. One of those little stick figures just visible in the glare was my youngest daughter Micheline, snorkelling with a friend. This was my dream holiday, we had flown up to Gladstone, taken a helicopter out to Heron Island, and now we were relishing four days of sunshine, wildlife, and relaxation. This was a wonderful 1997 Christmas gift from my Grandma as she approached her 103rd birthday!

Micheline had made a friend, and been out with her and her family each day. I had done most of the walks around the Island, and enjoyed watching the turtles, birds and other coral reef sights immensely. But I felt very lonely – very excluded from the family groups around me and the young couples enjoying each other. For the first time in my life I began to feel the pains of loneliness. It was a real physical feeling of anguish and despair. I had always been so self sufficient, busy, focused and organised, pouring my energies into my girls and their lives, as well as my work. Now I felt empty, half of a person somehow. But I put it all behind me as we travelled back home.

'Anyway,' I kept telling myself, 'it is silly to focus on my loneliness, as there is little I can do about it. After all, I've been diagnosed with a terminal illness, and the medical prognosis is at best for up to ten years of living at home with increasing levels of help, before needing to go into nursing home care.'

'But surely if I am feeling better supposedly because of prayers for my healing, shouldn't I really believe I am better and behave accordingly?' I carried on this conversation with myself over the days and weeks ahead.

'Well, maybe,' I lukewarmly agreed, 'and perhaps I should go out and socialise a bit more. But at the age of 49, where am I going to meet people?'

Church was the same group of friends, comfortable and secure. I was not meeting many new people, in a new environment. Maybe I needed to step out and challenge myself a bit more. But then, wasn't this being silly? Who gets better with dementia? Who tries new things when they have this disease? Who'd want to make friends with me?

It was my friend Liz MacKinlay, the priest and gerontological nursing lecturer who had persuaded me to write my first book, who encouraged me to consider going to study at St Mark's Theological College. I mused at the possibilities here – I would meet people for sure, and it would be a supportive and positive environment. I felt really challenged now. How could I sign up for a degree, nine years part time, when I was declining every day with dementia?

Alzheimer's is meant to take away your ability to learn new things, like getting to new places, meeting new people, doing new things. And here I was thinking about a degree!!!! The conversation in my head began again! 'But didn't I really believe I was getting better?'

Embarking on studies

One day in early February 1998, just a year after my surprising Heron Island experience of loneliness, I had dropped my daughter off at school, and was driving along a road in Canberra, one that leads across a bridge over the still grey waters of the lake. Just before the bridge, I realised that St Mark's College was just over the road.

It was a beautiful sunny day, I was in no hurry, and thought that maybe I would just pop in and find out about their courses. The lady at the desk gave me the information and then asked if I'd like to meet the registrar to find out more. 'OK,' I said, 'I'd like to know a bit more about how many units you have to do and in what areas, and how long it takes.' The registrar ushered me into her small, chaotic and paper-strewn office. I sat on the only chair that was not covered with papers.

She was enthusiastic, warm and welcoming. 'Courses are starting next week. Why don't you simply sign up now? I can get you in right away if you want. Here, take this form with you and you can drop it off later on today if you want to go ahead.' Looking at the form at home, I laughed out loud at the section that said 'Do you have any disabilities that might interfere with your studies?' Carefully I wrote in 'Alzheimer's Disease', thinking how ridiculous this would seem to the university administration. Maybe they would treat it as a student prank?

But I was worried. How would I cope trying to listen to lectures, absorbing new information, meeting new people, and doing essays on topics about which I knew nothing as yet? It was a great relief when each of the lecturers I met was kind, and asked what they could do to help me. They knew about my diagnosis, and about how I was trying to live positively each day, and to overcome my feelings of despair.

It was clear to them and to me that I could not hang onto new information for very long, but that I could interact with ideas, work on reading and taking notes, and try to prepare essays with lots of time. Many days I was simply not able to study – my brain was not focused, my head hurt, and my eyes somehow would not work properly. I needed clear lecture notes, time to read and absorb, and it was soon easy to see that I would cope better working in the distance education mode, with frequent visits to the College when I felt well enough to do so.

Meeting all these new people was wonderful, and I felt as if I was beginning to crawl out of my shell. It was stimulating to have new ideas, facts and issues being debated around me, to have challenges such as trying to write an essay, and to manage to get my increasingly limited brain space to absorb and process concepts that were totally new to me. I enjoyed the quiet of St Mark's library, with its smell of old paper, and its closely spaced high shelves full of tightly packed and catalogued books, which had been opened long ago by other students seeking information. I bought a new computer, and learnt how to use all its various functions. Searching the Internet became a passion, as did reading and discovering so much new information.

My studies went very well, and when my first essay was returned to me with a High Distinction I realised that the bits of my brain that were left were obviously still working very well indeed! Maybe my 'brain steroid' – my anti-dementia drug – was giving me an added advantage. It certainly was clearing the fog in my brain, and helping me to function, slowly but capably.

But still I had this medical diagnosis and prognosis hanging over me. I had been told the standard dementia script by the first neurologist I had seen: 'You have about five years till you become demented, then a few years after that in a nursing home till you die.' It was so hard to shake off this dismal prognosis, and to just take each day at a time, as my current neurologist was encouraging me to do. How could I believe in a rosy future, in completing the entire post-graduate diploma course? I was doing this part time, and I was certain I could not last the distance.

Going to the neurologist with Ianthe in May 1998 for the check up, and for the follow-up scans and tests in July, was a 'circuit breaker' for me. Either I was really improving, or maybe I was staying on a plateau without getting any worse, or feeling better was just a figment of my imagination. The neurologist would be able to see whether the prognosis was still as bad as it was the year before. This would really help me to believe that I had a future, one in which the prospect of actually gaining a new qualification was a possibility. I was happy to do as many tests as he wanted.

While undergoing all the tests in Sydney, I began to think 'What if I will last a lot longer and not get so sick so soon?' But this happy prospect of good health brought with it feelings of sadness, as then as I would have years and years alone to experience the pain of loneliness that I had felt – an almost physical feeling – whilst on Heron Island.

Wishful thinking, or a vision of the future?

I used to sit in my living room, teary and lonely. 'What a wimp!' I thought. 'How come this is the first time in my life that I have ever wanted a companion? What's wrong with me?' I think my girls sensed that I was not quite as content as usual with my own company, and for Mother's Day in 1998 they gave me a teddy bear. Certainly an improvement, but not quite the real thing!

That May/June, I was reading my daily bible study book.[8] I was astounded as before me was a series of meditations on loneliness. I sobbed my way through each of these, often praying passionately, and realising what fervent prayer really was. There I was, prone, weeping with the tissue box beside me. Thank goodness no one was at home to see me!

But then during one of these times of weeping and praying, I had this strange picture in my head, almost like a video clip, maybe some people might call it a vision. In this 'waking dream', I felt that I was in the passenger seat of my own car, with a pile of papers on my lap, the engine running and the driver's door open. Somehow I got the feeling that my life partner was going to get into the car, and that I had the maps on my lap, with which to help him in his ministry and our life together.

Well, I was sure this was just wishful thinking, of course. Maybe I had fallen asleep and had a dream. Wouldn't you? Anyway, I soon forgot all about this silly bit of fanciful thinking, and got on with my studies.

But the loneliness became stronger, the emptiness somehow more overwhelming, so I reviewed my life. Where was I going to make new friends, where was I going to meet people who might take me out for dinner or to the movies? Not at church, everyone was too busy and too protective of my health. Not at studies, everyone was focused on their work, and their very busy lives.

Meeting Paul

I had been at St Mark's College for a few months and things were going well. Now Ianthe was driving me from Canberra to Sydney for my check up with the neurologist. We chatted about this and that as the tarmac road hurtled beneath, and the bush landscape rolled past. Finally I managed to pluck up courage to really open up and share with her my feelings of loneliness. Soon I was sobbing my way through several tissues. I said how I was so shy and would find it very hard to meet anyone, as I was too afraid even to ask someone to come for a cup of coffee with me.

'I can't believe you, Mum. You always seem so sure of yourself. So in control. Surely you could simply ask someone to have coffee with you?'

'I could if it were a woman, but I would be literally shaking if it were a man,' I confessed. I talked about the possibility of joining an introductions agency, and wondered out loud if God could work through such an agency to find the right person for me.

Finally I was very bold, surprising myself and all my friends. Maybe it was really a sign of dementia to be this impulsive, to act this much out-of-character. But I managed to pluck up the courage to sign up to an introductions agency. In my prayers I made this deal with God, that if it was his will for me to be alone for the rest of this new life that I thought he had given me, then that was OK. However, if not, could he please work through this agency to find me the person he had chosen for me.

THE PHONE RANG loudly in the kitchen – it was the lady from the agency. 'We have a nice gentleman who we think you would like to meet. His name is Paul and he has been a diplomat for the Australian Government.' She told me he liked sailing, music, motorbikes and travelling. This sounded very intriguing. So I said 'OK, he can give me a ring on Friday evening.' The agency suggested we arrange a meeting somewhere in a public place for coffee or a walk.

I was so nervous on Friday evening, and when the phone rang, I picked it up hoping my fear could not be heard, as I said 'Hello, yes this is Christine.' We arranged to meet on the steps of the National Library for a walk by the lake, at 12 noon on Saturday.

The next day I felt ill with apprehension! I dressed in my purple trousers and silk jacket, woollen gloves and comfortable walking shoes. My hands were sticky and it felt difficult to breathe easily. It was a sunny but very chilly winter's day, with the sky a deep clear blue, as I drove into the Library car park wondering which car might be his.

I stood on the steps as this man about my age came towards me, smiling. He had blond reddish hair, glasses hiding his watery blue eyes, neatly trimmed beard, and a cord jacket and trousers. I was trying to take it all in. What was he like? Would he like me? Lots of thoughts filled my mind as he thrust a bunch of bright yellow daffodils into my hands. 'Hello,' he said, 'I'm Paul.'

I was overcome, not knowing whether to take off my gloves to shake his hand, where to put the flowers. Fumbling around in shyness, I thanked him for the flowers, stuffed my gloves in my pocket and shook his hand! Self-consciously we walked off together towards the still grey water of the lake, as I gripped tightly onto my bunch of flowers. We decided to lay the flowers on the nearby memorial to a girl who had recently been tragically killed in an accident there.

We started walking around the lake, talking about our lives, our children, our family life, where we had worked, where we had lived. Paul said he had a simple lunch in his backpack, and we decided to stop at a picnic spot just around the lake. He produced a blue seer-sucker table cloth from his backpack, laid it out on the picnic table and proceeded to lay out a magnificent spread of crusty bread, cheese, pickle, butter, plates, knives and even French wine and wine glasses! I was overcome.

Paul was so nice, that I felt terrible about *not* letting him know about my illness beforehand! I plucked up enough courage to tell him the whole truth about me, about my illness, expecting this to be the last time I would see this wonderful person. After all, who wants to date someone dying of a disease like Alzheimer's?

So sitting on the wooden bench in the chilly Canberra winter sun, I sipped my red wine, and told him all about my diagnosis with Alzheimer's Disease. I said that the doctors thought that I would need full nursing care in about five years, and would probably die a few years after that. Paul talked about his father dying of Alzheimer's, and did not seem at all put off by what I thought was bound to be the end of our relationship, when it had hardly begun.

We continued walking around the lake until the light started to dim, and the air became chilly and damp. Finally we decided to go back to our cars, realising that we both had sore feet and hoarse throats! As we dawdled at my car door, to say goodbye, I plucked up enough courage to ask Paul if he would like to see a movie I had wanted to see, but knew my girls did not want to go to. We arranged to meet again the next day and saw the movie.

As we sipped our hot coffee at a nearby café after the movie, I told Paul that I'd be away for a few days with my daughter, to visit my dear friend Leanne. I had spoken in my book about meeting Leanne every Friday evening for dinner, to commiserate and reflect on the past week.[9] She had now moved away to a farm south of Canberra, so the next day, Micheline and I boarded the bus for the six-hour trip. We had a wonderful time, sitting in front of a roaring log fire, walking in the beautiful countryside, tasting delicious red wines, and of course talking for hours, sharing all that had been happening in our lives. I told her about meeting Paul, about how lovely he was, and yet how I felt bewildered, bemused and perplexed, and wondered what to do.

When Micheline and I returned home, the answering machine was blinking insistently. I pushed the button and heard several messages from Paul, each one becoming more anxious as to when I might be coming home. Soon I plucked up courage to ring him, and he sounded delighted to hear my voice.

We saw each other a great deal those first few weeks, and of course now I can tell you that it was Paul, in his modest red car, who dropped me off at the bus station that cold day in early July to travel to Sydney for my tests.

A few weeks later we travelled together to Sydney to visit his family for his birthday. His mother greeted me warmly, and made me feel very welcome. We went with her to meet Paul's brother Ian and his wife, at a delightful Japanese restaurant nearby. I was so nervous. What would his brother think of me? But soon I felt right at home, as we chatted away over sushi and tempura. As we said our goodbyes in front of the restaurant, Ian gave me a big hug and said 'Welcome to the family.' I was overwhelmed. That night, before going to bed, I gave Paul his first big hug from me, and wished him a very happy birthday. My emotions were in turmoil!

But over the next few weeks I realised there was a large part of my life I could not really share wholeheartedly with Paul. I was a strong Christian, with a supportive church family. I went regularly to church and read my bible, and my faith had sustained me through so much.

Paul believed that God probably existed, and he went to church at Christmas and at Easter. His faith journey was very different.

Finally I suggested that Paul go back to the agency – much to the astonishment of my girls who knew how much I liked him! Ostensibly I said it was because I was only his first introduction, and there must be lots of lovely ladies waiting to meet him, so it did not seem fair to him to only meet me, someone who had Alzheimer's Disease. Paul and I had often joked about the agency being the Old Dog's Home, and that we were like a couple of lost old dogs who were looking for a good home. Back to the Old Dog's Home Paul went! He got a list of names from the agency, but never got to ring them!

Instead, my phone rang, insistently and loudly on the following Monday morning. It was Paul. 'I want to marry you, and take care of you, as I think I have been told to look after you.'

I gulped, this was all too much to take in, we had only known each other a few weeks! I said 'Perhaps you could come over for lunch and we could have a chat?' I put the phone down, my mind reeling. Yes, Paul was lovely, but this was so fast, so sudden, so unexpected. And just who was it who had been speaking to him about taking care of me?

He came rushing in that lunchtime, a big grin on his face, eyes shining, face beaming with delight. He started to tell me about the previous evening, when he had been sitting in his bed, ready to go to sleep. Suddenly the room was full of this vivid movie, perhaps like a waking dream. He was amazed as he saw us riding together on a motor bike, with a side car. We got off to look at the sunset, and a towering shimmering being got out of the side car. This shimmering being then calmly put me on the back of the bike, turned around and said to Paul, in a quiet, firm yet gentle voice, 'I will take care of her now', and rode off into the sunset with me.

Paul felt strongly that this vision, or whatever it was, meant that he had been told to look after me until I died, when I would be taken safely away. Medically that could be in a few years time. He became a Christian, joined me at church each Sunday and came to my bible study group, and began a rapid learning curve of living joyfully in faith as part of the family of Christ. And the poet in him began to flow, to burst out of him like a release of love and joy!

First Paul wrote this poem about how it did not matter if we only had a few precious years together, before I declined and died with dementia.

How long

How long do we have before our candle's out?
Forty, ten years, five, one?
Six months, a week, a day – too short sure!
But I'd not complain. Better one day than none.

Then he wrote this next poem about how he would be there for me until I died with dementia, and that when he in time died, we would be together again.

When you lie down to sleep

When you lie down to sleep
I'll hold your hand.
Soft breathe, calm heart, content.
When you lie down last to sleep
Soft breathe your last on the Valley floor
I'll hold your hand
Not content until
My heart slow stops
Then content we're one once more.

Soon the muse and the poet were spending a lot of time together. Paul came round for breakfast, lunch and dinner, only going away to work and sleep. It was as if he didn't want to waste any time, a precious commodity for me. We packed a great deal of talking, of sharing, into just a few months.

It was a time during which my daughters needed to adjust to this new person, competing for this precious time with their mother who was battling a terminal illness. It was not at all easy for them, especially for Micheline who was living with me at the time. We had become very close, just the two of us, after her sisters had left to go to university.

A few months after Paul and I had met, when Ianthe and Rhiannon were home, we all sat around the dining table, after eating our Sunday roast dinner. Paul stood up and gave a little speech to my girls, in which he promised that the only hand he would ever raise to me would be one to help. There were a few teary eyes around the table that day, as the girls and I realised his sincerity and willingness to begin this journey alongside us, the dance with dementia.

Vision becomes reality!

The phone rang, while Paul and I were busily preparing a meal together one evening in September 1998. I picked it up and it was the neurologist with the results of all those tests in May and in July.

'I've looked at the scans, and compared them with those that were taken three years ago now. I've also examined the psychometric follow-up tests.' He said, 'The pattern does not seem to be typical of Alzheimer's, and is more like a fronto-temporal dementia. Also from what I have seen in your functioning, and the differences in the various scans taken now and back in 1995, it does appear as if the deterioration is glacially slow.'

I was speechless! I managed to squeak 'Does this mean I might live long enough to see my girls graduate, to see any grandchildren? Could I last another 10 years or more?'

He quietly replied, 'I don't see why not, given the current rate of decline, and your ability to keep functioning.'

We danced around my kitchen at this news! We would have more time together that either of us had dreamed could be possible.

A FEW WEEKS later, I drove my little green car to Paul's house, as we planned to go together that evening to a sailing club meeting. We agreed to go together in my car, and as I was tired, Paul would drive.

Paul sat in the car, started the engine, and studied the maps to work out where the meeting was. But then he suddenly remembered that some papers were still in his house, so he gave me the maps, leapt out of the car, left the door open, and the engine running, and dashed off to his house.

I had forgotten my strange vision up until that time – but it certainly came back vividly at that moment. There I was, in the passenger seat of my car, engine running, driver's door open, and a pile of papers on my lap. I felt quite wobbly inside, with shivers down my spine. Tentatively, I shared this with Paul as we drove to the meeting.

IN JULY 1999, I was sitting in my counselling class at St Mark's, with my colleagues, wondering why Paul wanted to meet me there for lunch that day. Just an hour later, I walked back into my next class, with my world changed forever, and I started to tell them why I looked so radiant.

Paul had led me by the hand into the small, slate-floored chapel. We had sat quietly on the low wooden bench, gazing out of the beautiful glass window, with its frosted design of a cross. Beyond the glass pane was a swathe of moist green grass, dappled with the shadows of a large tree, where small birds chirped and flurried. In the distance was the calm water of the lake.

Paul dropped to his knees, took out a small box, and said 'Christine Eva Boden, will you marry me?' I was speechless and overcome. All I could manage was a breathless 'Yes'. I put on the ring, a large blue topaz that his mother had bought many years ago in Brazil, when she travelled there with his father to visit Paul. It was a very special gift to us, carrying memories of his father, and representing his mother's love and acceptance.

What followed was a frenetic time of organising by my church family, as we planned to get married just a month later. The love they showed us was amazing. All the organising, the flowers, the invitations, all the arrangements were taken care of, so a great weight of worry and anxiety was lifted from me. All I had to do was organise my dress.

Why the rush? Not only were we both conscious of our time together being precious, but we had talked to my mum in England about arrangements. She was unable to come, because of her health, but she really wanted my brother-in-law, Ivor, to give me away on behalf of my father, who had died the year before I met Paul. And my sister and Ivor, who lived in Hong Kong, were able to come across to Australia with their boys only if we were able to set a date sometime in the last two weeks of August.

We managed to organise the wedding for 21 August 1999. It was a warm sunny winter's day, and the church was filled with family, friends and relatives for the celebration. As I got out of the car with Ivor, and arranged my gold dress, I tried to hold my creamy orchids steady despite my shaking hands. I was so nervous! All morning I had busied myself, getting fresh flowers in my hair, make-up on, and my dress. Flowers had arrived from friends, so the house was filled with their delicate scent. All too soon, Ivor was there with the white wedding car, with its white ribbons.

At the door of the church, Ivor took my shaking hand, speaking to me gently, and encouraging me. Then he led me slowly up the aisle, through the lines of people standing, and there was Paul waiting for me at the altar, grinning with his white silk jacket and gold cummerbund. Our minister guided us through a delightful celebration in which we exchanged our vows, and shared our joy, our faith and our hope with friends and family.

A very special moment in the wedding ceremony was when we washed each other's feet, using a thick new fluffy white towel, and a basin of warm water. We wanted to demonstrate how we would be caring for each other's needs in love, like the description of Jesus washing his friends' feet. It was deeply touching for our friends and family, knowing the journey that we were to make together, this journey with dementia.

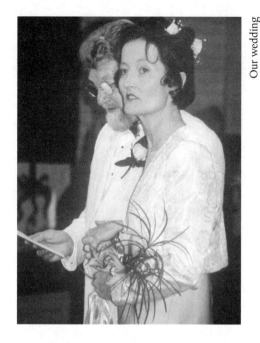

Our wedding

My friends said 'We were all so overjoyed! Just four years ago we thought we would lose you to Alzheimer's Disease. Now you are still here, and getting married to such a lovely man. What a miracle!' Each day since that crisp sunny August afternoon does seem like a true miracle to me – not only am I better than I could have hoped for, but I now have a loving husband who shares my strong faith. Even just a few years ago, I could not have dreamed any of this was possible.

2

'Coming Out'
With Dementia

Challenging the stereotype

It took me three years before I could speak openly about my diagnosis, overcoming the hopelessness and depression that exacerbated my dementia and took me on a downward spiral of dysfunction. Climbing back from this pit of despair had been a struggle, one in which my faith had sustained me, as well as the prayers of my friends.

It was all too easy to believe the stereotype of dementia, of the late stages of the disease, of being unable to recognise anyone and of being unable to speak. It was a constant battle to overcome the fear of these later stages that were so prominently the picture everyone had of dementia. No one seemed to talk about the long journey beforehand, between diagnosis and the end stage – the journey of living with dementia each day.

The publication of my book catapulted me reluctantly into the public eye in mid 1998, as someone with dementia who could still speak, and who was also prepared to talk openly about this disease and what it felt like to be on the journey from diagnosis to death. It was the first time anyone in Australia had 'owned up' to having dementia. I had 'come out', disclosing my disease, rather like those with AIDS must feel, brave enough to admit to a disease that people dread. Dementia was a shameful disease, to be feared or denied, not one to be acknowledged and battled with.

The myths and fears about dementia – the stereotype of someone in the later stages of the diseases that cause dementia – give rise to stigma which isolates us. You say we do not remember, so we cannot understand. We do not know, so it is OK to distance yourself from us. And you treat us with fear and dread. We cannot work, we cannot drive, we cannot contribute to society. I am watched carefully for signs of odd words or behaviour, my opinion is no longer sought, and I am thought to lack insight, so it does not matter that I am excluded.

But if I do have insight, and can speak clearly or write about my experiences, then I am said to lack credibility as a true representative of people with dementia. Why is this so? Maybe it is because the stereo-type, and the stigma, are based on the end stages of dementia. But dementia is not just an end stage, it is a journey, from diagnosis to death, and there are many steps along the way. My battle for credibility in making this journey was at first a lonely one.

Finding help and support

In October 1995, I was still reeling from the shock of just having been diagnosed with Alzheimer's Disease. I picked up the phone tentatively and managed to ring the number for the Alzheimer's Association. 'I'd like some information about being diagnosed with Alzheimer's Disease, please.'

The voice on the other end of the phone said 'Who is it that you are caring for, your mother or father? Husband?' I gulped, and said in a very small voice 'Actually, it's me who has been diagnosed. Is there anything you have for people with dementia?' The response was that there was really very little available that would be suitable, as most material was directed towards the carer, who was supposedly at home looking after me, in my incapacity and my inability to communicate. I put down the phone, feeling cast adrift. The nearest I had to a 'carer' was my eldest daughter, and she was only 19 years old, and over 300 km away at university in Sydney!

I felt as if I had been abandoned by the very organisation I thought had been set up to help me. Surely if I had cancer and had rung up the cancer society, they would not have suggested that only my family could have help?

I STRUGGLED ON as best I could, wrote my book, and dealt with the emotional, psychological pain of this new life I was facing, in which Alzheimer's Disease seemed to dominate. But by May 1998, I had dispatched my book to the publishers, was studying at St Mark's, and was beginning to feel well enough to try again, to approach the Alzheimer's Association to ask for help for people with dementia. I was so concerned that by only helping carers, those of us living on our own were being left without help, struggling with our emotions, the sense of being alone, the only one with this terrible disease, and being too ashamed to tell anyone about it.

So I plucked up courage to go and find the offices of the local Alzheimer's Association. I had a false start, turning up at a dementia library, finding very little there apart from a few books and a junior office member. There was *no way* I was going to own up to the fact that I was a person with dementia. But the people there, assuming I was a carer of someone of course, gave me the address of the ACT Alzheimer's Association

A few days later, a beautiful sunny, warm May morning, I received the galley proofs of my first book. They looked great! Maybe they would act as a 'prop' for talking to someone at the Association, maybe they would prove I was someone with dementia, give me the necessary credentials somehow?

With my proofs in hand, I managed to find the offices of the ACT Alzheimer's Association, above a bank in a shopping centre in Canberra. As I walked up the stairs, and pushed the door open, I felt anxious and worried about what to say. Would they believe I was a person with dementia? After all, I could speak, so maybe I was a carer. But maybe the galley proofs would prove I had Alzheimer's Disease? All these thoughts were swirling around in my head, as the phones rang insistently, and the photocopier clunked and clicked. A lovely friendly lady, with red hair, vivid green dress, and a bright cheerful personality, welcomed me. She said she was delighted to meet me, and made me feel accepted as someone struggling with dementia, someone who needed support.

She put the answering machine on, and sat me down in a comfy chair with a cup of tea. I found out that her name was Michelle McGrath, and that she had just started as the Executive Director, volunteering her time to establish help for people with dementia and their families.

I told Michelle about being diagnosed with Alzheimer's Disease, and about writing my book. I said, 'People with dementia need help too. Could you maybe identify a few other people who have been diagnosed with dementia and who might want to meet together regularly to chat over a cup of tea?' Later I found out that this was a timely approach, as the Association had been considering its services for people with dementia, not just for carers.

The 'friends group', as we called it, was set up in June 1998, for four of us ladies with dementia, and Michelle was always there smiling, chatty, remembering how we liked our tea, and facilitating our discussions. Her enthusiasm and openness made each one of us feel valued and accepted for who we were, despite our illness. We went out together for shopping, for coffee, and developed a close friendship, sharing some important emotions of despair, depression, anger and confusion.

I remember that one day, Nora (not her real name), who was always immaculately dressed and had her nails manicured and painted, said, 'I had a big argument at the weekend with my husband who wouldn't move the boxes in front of the car because he said there were no boxes there.' We chatted about this for a while, and then I gently said, 'Some of us with dementia see things other people don't see. I know that last year I had some terrible times like that.' She looked amazed, and said, 'Do you mean the boxes I saw were not real?' She pondered a bit more and went on, 'My poor husband, I really shouted at him about those boxes. Maybe they weren't really there at all.'

A few weeks later, she said she was frightened of what seemed to look like tigers lurking in the back of her wardrobe. When I visited her, I realised there was a mirror at the back of her walk-in wardrobe which could reflect things and make them look very scary, especially without the light on. We spoke to her husband about this, so that he could make sure that maybe the mirror was covered up and the light always on.

I went to visit Helen (again, not her real name) at home a few months after our group had started. She stayed at home while her husband went to work. Helen said she often felt lost, even in her own home. It was not really a matter of losing her way, but losing herself somehow, she said. She knew the house was there all around her and she could look down and see her body there, but somehow in her head, there was no sense of being a person existing in this space. Helen said it was worse when she was by herself, but when her husband, care worker or friends were there relating to her, she seemed to come back from somewhere where she had been lost. Maybe they acted like a mirror for her, reflecting her existence, reaffirming her personhood.

During the next six months, I continued to go to my friends group, as my new life was unfolding with Paul. I shared with them my hopes and fears for the future. Soon Paul became interested in helping with the Alzheimer's Association. By the beginning of 1999, he was able to have two days free each week, and so offered to help the Association to set up another group as well. We met in a community centre, sharing cups of tea or coffee, and sometimes we would have outings or picnics.

Often we had circular discussions, as we could not remember what we had just said, so a frequent comment was 'I may have told you this before, but...!' There was a lot of humour, a lot of openness, and a feeling of all being in this together.

All of our friends from the groups were invited to our wedding, to share in our joy. It was wonderful! I remember Eric (not his real name) rushing in a little late, just as I was getting out of the wedding car. He said to me 'Oh, how lovely you look, and what a surprise to see you here!' Nora was sitting in her wheelchair, smiling, and greeted me warmly after the service. In our group a few weeks later, she said I looked lovely going down the aisle, in my gold dress. But then, just a few sentences later, she said she was not there. As we gently talked about this, she pointed to her head, and tearfully expressed her aware-ness that up there, in her head, she had not been there. I choked up with tears as I hugged her.

With Michelle, we then organised a workshop in 1999, for people with dementia and their families. We wanted to see whether having these groups was helping families to cope. We hoped to identify com-munication problems, so we held two concurrent sessions: one for people with dementia and one for their family members. The same questions were asked of both groups. At the end, both groups came together and each group reported their responses to our questions, and there was a great deal of humour and enjoyment during this session.

The first question asked was: 'Do you think "your family/you" understand what the person with dementia is feeling?' A common thread in responses from the people with dementia was while their family was the most important thing in their lives, the family didn't really understand what it was like not to remember the most ordinary, everyday things. Yes, we all agreed it was a great idea to have a diary, but sometimes, a lot of the time you had to be reminded to look in the diary! We all agreed and were grateful to have the support of our loving families, but what we all wanted was to be listened to, to be asked what our wishes were.

One person told the story of how, literally days after his diagnosis, his wife started to do every single thing for him. The thing that irri-tated him most was the way she laid out his clothes for him every morning as if he were a little boy. He felt he couldn't tell her because that would upset her, but he became so frustrated that he began to get angry and shout at his wife. His wife and family of course were dis-traught, and the anxiety levels of both the person with dementia and his family increased to such a point that outside intervention was required. All this anxiety because the person with dementia didn't want to hurt his wife's feelings, and his wife of course thought she was doing the right thing, but she didn't ever ask.

When we asked people what difference coming to the group had made, all the answers were very positive. For example, Jack (not his real name), who was in his 70s and always happy to make cups of coffee, said, 'This is the happiest I have been for a very long time, it's like a big happy family. I feel 100 per cent better and wouldn't know what to do otherwise. I have more chance to talk, and no one is irritated – everyone understands and listens. We are all in the same boat.'

Peter (not his real name) said, 'I love this room, it is like my child-hood cubby house, I can do and say anything in this room and nobody will get upset or offended.'

Leanne (not her real name), who was always smartly dressed and ready to go when we arrived to take her to the group, was very careful getting the words right before she gave her answer. She had been a teacher and one of her main concerns was losing her vocabulary. Leanne said, 'I look forward to it each week – though I forget the day! Everyone has a chance to talk – we converse a lot. Being part of the group has made it easier to live with my disease. It is very helpful, as I need information to pass onto my family.'

Janet (not her real name) had not been on outings, nor had friends to visit since being diagnosed. She had been reluctant to come to the group at first, but after the first meeting she kept asking when the next one would be held. She did not want to miss out! Janet told the group, 'I love going out, having coffee, shopping, going to the movies with a group of like-minded friends. A group of ordinary people doing ordinary things together. We are normal again!'

When we asked if people wanted to carry on being in a group, all of them said yes. Leanne said, 'Yes – no "ifs" or "buts", I'd miss it if I could not come.' And Janet said, 'Just try to stop me!'

We then asked the families what they thought. Margaret (not her real name) said: 'Yes – he is more outgoing and not as withdrawn as before. He seems brighter, happier and more chatty on the group day, and has more conversation. Why not spend money on the people themselves, not afternoon teas etc. for carers?'

Paula (not her real name) talked of her husband enjoying himself. 'He comes back refreshed, and that in itself takes the pressure off me. I get time out while he is at this meeting and he comes back more relaxed.'

Alexander (not his real name) commented 'It has been positive, and provided a focus. She looks forward to it and enjoys talking about it.'

All the families agreed that these changes had happened within about three or four meetings. We wanted to check with the agency that had referred people to the group, to see if the changes that we saw could be observed more objectively. The worker was asked to come to lunch with the group and see if any changes could be observed. She said:

> When I shared the barbecue lunch with this group a few months after I had assessed the clients I was struck most of all by the sheer 'normality' of the event. This is not meant in any patronising or condescending way. In fact it was clearly evident that no one was being patronised or cared for; rather there was a sense of mutual care and support and sharing and most of all joy, good humour and firmly established bonds.
>
> The second most striking change in all of the people (whom I had visited at home previously) was their relaxed facial expressions and posture. The tension and the sense of hopelessness and defeat that I had felt were no longer in evidence. No doubt, they still have many moments of feeling these things, but at least they now have the opportunity to deal with some of these feelings in a safe environment with other people who know exactly what they are talking about.

Her words resonated with me, as they very much captured my feelings. The hopelessness and despair that I had felt after diagnosis were diminishing as I shared my feelings with others. I no longer felt alone, and knew that the Association, particularly Michelle, was there to help me. I was making new friends and going on outings, and I felt as if I was helping, doing something worthwhile. I felt valued, and given back my human dignity and respect.

During that year I relaxed into this newfound safety net of support, and put my energies into helping out at the Association. But a rude shock awaited me.

Battling the stereotype – if I can speak then I do not have dementia!

We were enjoying a dinner during the national conference in Perth, just a month after our wedding. It was September 1999. I had spoken at a plenary session on the last day about my experiences as a person with dementia, and was tired yet happy to be involved and included, as someone struggling with this terminal illness, who was trying to reach out and help others understand what it was like.

At a nearby table, the Executive Director of one of the other State Associations said, 'But she lacks credibility as a person with dementia.' He was questioning whether I really could speak on behalf of people with dementia. I did not fit his stereotype of someone in the later stages. I was devastated. In what way did I lack credibility? Did he think I was faking it in some way? Why would I lie about having this illness that everyone feared and was ashamed of?

The next morning, there was a meeting to discuss support groups for people in the early stages of dementia, and I joined this small meeting in a sunny glass-walled room at the motel where we were staying. A lady there made it quite clear that she didn't want me there. She found it too difficult to talk to someone with dementia, because her husband had a similar diagnosis to me, and yet was unable to communicate. She found it far too confronting and emotional, so said things to me, and about me, that I found were so hurtful, so much like what had been happening in terms of no one believing that I really was struggling with this disease.

I left the meeting in tears, and still I remember the pain of that time, yet it made me even more determined to change this prevailing attitude that if I could speak, I did not have dementia.

THIS CONTINUING BATTLE to overcome such negative attitudes adds to my struggle with my illness. My diagnosis was questioned just the other day, when I was interviewed by a journalist from the USA. My diagnosis, she said, was nine years ago. It was no longer Alzheimer's, but something else. The subtext of her question was 'Maybe you don't really have dementia, maybe you can't really represent people with Alzheimer's Disease, who have the real thing.'

I tried to explain that the word dementia is an 'umbrella' term, covering a number of diseases with similar symptoms caused by brain damage. These symptoms include confusion, memory loss, speech and other language problems. I said that we accept that the word cancer is used for a number of different types of disease with similar symptoms caused by uncontrolled cell growth. Whether I have Alzheimer's Disease, vascular dementia, Lewy Body dementia or fronto-temporal dementia, I will still have similar symptoms caused by brain damage, and be suffering from a terminal illness for which there is no cure.

But the fact that I am still here, speaking out, baffles those who have this stereotype of someone in the late stages. If I can speak, I am not sick. This is the big dilemma, the 'Catch 22' of dementia.

I am often asked whether I really have dementia, my diagnosis is repeatedly questioned. But if I had gone public with, say, a diagnosis of breast cancer, would my diagnosis then be questioned? Would people want to see the lump, see the scars, receive proof of my illness? What is it about dementia that makes people demand proof if I can speak about my illness? Those in the late stages are the only ones with credibility, it seems. But after diagnosis, there is usually a journey of several years, in which we are battling the decline. And in this journey many of us can still speak.

All of us travelling this journey have a right to be heard, to be listened to, and to be regarded with respect. There is no time to lose to hear our voice as we struggle to communicate.

THERE IS A commonly held view, too, that the various stages of our journey can be categorised neatly into compartments, and that each of us can be carefully assessed and fitted into one of these categories.

I recall in 2003 sharing the podium at an international conference with a famous scientist, who has spent his career developing these descriptors. There were three of us on the stage, and he spoke first, I was to go next. He showed slide after slide, of graphs and tables describing what exactly we people with dementia could be expected to be like at each stage of our dementia, what we would no longer be able to do, and how we should be treated according to our step-by-step decline on this carefully described path. He sat down and I walked across to the lectern.

I didn't really know where to start, after such a scientific analysis of me and my disease, so I simply said 'I don't know where I fit on the stages you have just heard about. There are lots of things I can't do now, but there are others that I can still do, although perhaps you would not expect me to be able to, according to the charts you have just seen.' My talk was a personal one, about being diagnosed with dementia, what it felt like to be labelled, to be given this medical script of decline in a certain time, and how I was still there despite all of this expectation. The third speaker threw away his notes, and did a masterful job at summarising the scientific and personal perspectives that the audience had just heard!

I am an individual, with a disease of my brain, the part of my body that is very much influenced by my personality, by my attitude. Certainly the disease is affecting me, steadily taking away more and more of my ability, but surely my individuality means it is going to be hard to categorise my decline so easily and with such confidence. And such charts and graphs and stages deny me my individuality, stripping me of any credibility at still being able to speak after years of living the journey of dementia.

We often hear of cancer survivors, people who have defied the odds by lasting much longer than doctors have expected them too. And we applaud their bravery, their courage, in this struggle to survive. But when we people with dementia don't decline as quickly as you think we should, or seem to last longer and speak out for longer and to be active, then you question our diagnosis.

Why is this so? Why can't you cheer the dementia survivors? Maybe many of us would survive better and longer if we did not have to battle against the stereotype of dementia. Maybe many of us find it easier to give up and act like you expect us to, not speaking much or really 'being there'.

Meeting my 'cyber' friends

I felt very alone, after that fateful dinner in Perth in 1999, when I realised that my battle with dementia was going to lead to repeated questioning of my diagnosis. But this feeling of being the only one with dementia able to speak and to challenge the accepted view of rapid decline into incoherence would all change in March 2000, when I got a phone call from my dear friend in the Sydney Alzheimer's Association library. She said 'There is a man in the US, Morris Friedell, who has Alzheimer's who has bought your book from us over the Internet. He'd like to get in touch with you. Would it be all right for me to give him your email address?'

I agreed, and over the next few months, I found out about a new Internet support group that Morris' friend Laura Smith had set up, called Coping With Personal Memory Loss. By the time of World Alzheimer's Day that year, when a few of them gathered together for a memory walk in the USA, this group became the Dementia Advocacy and Support Network (DASN).

It was wonderful to get emails regularly from friends in the USA and in Canada who also had a diagnosis of dementia, and yet like me were still able to communicate, willing to speak out, and wanting to challenge the accepted view of the late stages of the disease. Most of us were taking anti-dementia drugs, and we were not willing to accept being categorised into a medical model of decline according to set stages.

But maybe it was all too easy to hide behind our computer screens and talk to each other about how we felt. How were we going to change the attitudes we faced, those charts that said we had to decline, otherwise we were not really people with dementia? How were we going to challenge the idea of being the 'patient' or the 'sufferer', and let the world know we were individuals each struggling with a terminal illness?

Local and national advocacy

Michelle, our local Alzheimer's Association director, encouraged us to become involved in all the association activities. Soon she had co-opted Paul to the committee, as the President, and before very long, I had been elected to the management committee.

It was amazing to be involved in such a way, despite the stereotype of being a person with dementia, supposedly lacking capacity for such involvement. It certainly challenged a few people. But whenever my capacity was questioned, I said 'I am happy to do a mini mental status examination, as long as everyone else on this committee also does one.' This created some nervous laughter – no one was prepared to volunteer for this!

For me, the beginning of a long journey to change attitudes beyond our local region, together with my 'cyber friends in advocacy' in DASN, began in March 2001.

Taking the first step

We stood anxiously at the top of the air-bridge as the plane taxied in to Canberra airport. It was a sunny, but chilly day in late March. The leaves were a vivid display of autumn colour, as we drove to the airport that morning.

What would he look like? Would we recognize him? It had all started as a journey into cyberspace. I had seen Morris' photo on his web site, so I hoped we would recognise him. But there he was, just as I had imagined him, a small dark-grey haired 'professor' dragging behind him a large suitcase, which turned out to be full of books!

We had an inspiring week. Morris and I had long talks about the meaning of our individuality, reflecting on the atypical course of everyone's dementia, and discussing our struggle to be heard. We were grabbing snatches of thought and creativity in our intermittent bursts of energy, then fading into tiredness and blankness in-between.

Paul cooked and served meals, drove us around to see the autumnal colours, and smiled at our sputtering bursts of meteoric energy, followed by blank spaces of exhaustion. He laughed, and said 'I feel like Freud's wife when Einstein came to dinner, when I overhear you two talking about the meaning of life and death while I am in the kitchen!'

A few days of relaxing, and talking, and then we drove into the city of Canberra, for the national conference, where Morris and I were to give a joint plenary address.

I was exhausted. I had spent months preparing the talk, using PowerPoint for the first time, and incorporating both of our thoughts and ideas in a set of slides, exchanging numerous emails with Morris as we developed our presentation. Also we had been preparing material for special sessions for a dozen people with dementia from all over Australia who were attending this national conference. It was the first time in Australia, and perhaps in the world, that people with dementia were welcomed and encouraged to be active participants in a national conference.

I had spoken to each of these people on the phone. But several times I had to first explain to the spouse that I really wanted to speak to the person with dementia, because it was their views that were being sought, and their attendance at the conference being supported and encouraged. It was almost as if the person with dementia in that home was invisible, not allowed to come to the phone, no longer valued for their insights.

At the venue, Morris and I looked around the quiet room for these special sessions, with its comfy chairs, coffee and tea, and agreed it was a wonderful haven of rest during the busy conference. Both of us were to use it frequently over the next few days, to retreat from the bustle, and have some 'brain time-out', to restore our energy each time we faded with exhaustion.

For the first 'getting to know you' session, we stood anxiously at the door, to welcome each person as they came in. Carers hovered, not wanting to leave, and seemed very reluctant to let the person with dementia go in by themselves. It almost seemed as if they wondered why we would bother to listen to them, and whether they would be safe. Certainly they did not believe that we too were living with dementia.

In our final session, we were joined by the National Executive Director, Glenn Rees, as well as the President, Dr Robert Yeoh, of the Australian Alzheimer's Association, who both listened carefully and questioned us about our thoughts on what the Association was doing. As people with dementia, we were being validated and respected. The Executive Director is a quietly spoken, tall man, with a gentle unassuming manner, who had been only recently appointed. He had been very supportive, and made me feel very hopeful at the prospect of people with dementia being heard and being included. The President was a much shorter man, with a very welcoming smile. He is a doctor with a passion for helping families coping with dementia. They both made us feel that our views were being heard, and their willingness to listen gave us hope that people with dementia might be able to play a role within the life of the Association. The Consumer Focus Report which we produced is published by Alzheimer's Australia.[10]

The next day, Morris and I nervously walked up the steps to the platform, in front of a huge audience, hidden behind the lights that shone in our eyes. Paul and I had just spent a few hours with Morris, in the quiet room, helping him practice the speech, to read the words we had written, and to look up at the audience every now and then. Now I was to lead off our presentation, and then Morris would speak, in this plenary session on the final day of the conference.

Our slides spoke of the 'toxic power of the pointing-bone' of diagnosis. I described how it seems as if our world has come to an end, when we experience a defeat of spirit and of hope. We feel extreme fear of further loss, and dread what the future holds.

I quoted from an email of our friend Carole Mulliken on DASN, when she said 'The day before our diagnosis, we each could be vital and intimate partners in our personal relationships. The day after we had become a liability, like a pet, a mortgage or yesterday's laundry.'[11]

Morris had been a sociology professor, I had been a senior public servant. But overnight each of us had become simply another case of dementia. We were expected to withdraw from the world's stage and be assigned only the smallest walk-on parts. For me it seemed as if from then on I would only ever be allowed to function with my 'carer' in attendance. How come so much had changed overnight?

When Morris stood up to speak, he said:

> Our brain scans symbolise the moment of diagnosis, when our lives changed forever. By giving this talk, and functioning in this context, we are challenging the view that the person with dementia must lack insight, ability or judgement. You may be tempted to think that we are somehow misdiagnosed or the disease hasn't hit us, or that our ability to function here is so exceptional that it is irrelevant to other persons with dementia.
>
> But what if we were young persons who had suffered head impact in a motor accident and had analogous diffuse brain damage? And suppose we had rich and loving parents who sent us to top-notch rehabilitation programs and nourished us with vital hope that we could recover rich and productive lives. Our success then would not be so strange.

By this time in our joint presentation, the serried rows of heads watching us were motionless, nothing moved, and you could have heard a pin drop. Paul, who was sitting high up, in a back row, said he could see white tissues all around the rows of people below him, as moist eyes were dabbed, and our words reached into hearts and minds.

Morris went on to say:

> All that is given to persons with dementia is 'hospice in slow motion'. We reject this. There is life after a diagnosis of dementia, for both ourselves and our families. The toxic lie is that our abnormal brains make us biologically inferior.

Haven't I heard about 'biological inferiority' somewhere
before? The Nazis…the Holocaust.

Speaking as a Jew, these words were very powerful, and more white
tissues rustled and flurried around the audience as Morris carried on:

> We need to live a contradiction to the toxic lie of dementia –
> to live an exorcism, as it were, countering the curse of the
> pointing-bone of diagnosis. We can be guided to simple ther-
> apeutic behaviours in which failure is unlikely, and through
> which we can start to recover our shattered sense of compe-
> tence. We can discover ways of participating in life through
> giving and caring which restore our sense of value and
> meaning. Thus strengthened we find that again we can face
> and surmount challenges, and affirm our courage and dignity.

Now, as I reflect on Morris' words, and reproduce them here, I realise
how they truly marked a 'sea-change'. They were the beginning of
speaking out with power and dignity, to challenge current attitudes
and to look with hope to a new future. The ripple effect of his words
were to reach well beyond Canberra, to Australia, and beyond. He
said:

> It's as if we are bilingual or bicultural. Exiled from our past
> lifestyle we have lots of time to deeply and creatively relate.
> And we are conscious of the preciousness of our brief sojourn
> on earth. Having survived trauma, we know our strength. Our
> cognition may be fading, but we can draw on powerful
> resources – our emotions and our spirituality – to relate to
> you. Having been where you are, we can reach out across the
> divide to touch you in a new way.

He spoke of how we in DASN knew what it feels like to have the 'de-
generating sense of nobodiness' that Martin Luther King described as
affecting black Americans. Morris talked of how the Dementia
Advocacy and Support Network International (DASNI) aspired to
change views, quoting King, who had encouraged his people to

'protest courageously and yet with dignity and Christian love', qualities which would be remembered by future generations.[12]

I then walked to the lectern, feeling inadequate to follow on from this powerful message, but concluded our joint presentation by saying:

> As dementia survivors, we know both the world of 'normals' and that of dementia intimately, and we have weathered an extraordinary transition. By making this presentation, we are claiming our full participation in cultural life, and making a stand for all people with cognitive limitations. Morris and I are in solidarity as Christian and Jew, as persons with Alzheimer's and fronto-temporal dementia, as Australian and American.
>
> We seek to work towards transforming our culture to one honouring human dignity – or humankind as created in the divine image. Let's be companions together on this journey towards dementia survival with dignity.[13]

I sat down next to Morris, relieved, and tired.

We were puzzled, because the chair of our session tugged us both to the front of the stage. We realized that the applause was continuing. I peered into the glare of the lights and realised the entire audience was standing up clapping. Morris and I were overcome, and we nervously acknowledged this overwhelming support.

At the end of the conference, people with dementia came to the microphone and spoke, saying things like 'I have never spoken publicly about having dementia before.' They were crying as they shared how they felt, and how this conference had made them feel welcomed and affirmed.

It was the beginning of a long journey, that was to take us round the world in cyberspace, as well as face to face. The first step towards changing attitudes towards people with dementia had been launched in the autumn colours of Canberra. The next step was to take place in the summer warmth of Montana.

Going global

Paul had organised a trip in July that would take us to New Zealand for a few days rest, then to Montana for a week of work with our DASNI friends. After that, we would be going to Toronto to meet with the Canadian Alzheimer's Society, and on to London to meet with Alzheimer's Disease International (ADI). On the way home we planned to go to Berlin to a friend of mine for a day or so, then Poland, where Paul wanted to stay a few days to show me where he once lived.

All in all, it was going to be a whirlwind tour, with very little rest or downtime, and lots of work, papers to write and to print out, people to meet and to talk to. I was exhausted at the thought of going, but so grateful to the pharmaceutical company that sponsored our tickets to go to Montana and London.

Teddy's world travels

My youngest daughter, Micheline, came round to say goodbye, before we left on our long journey. She gave me a carefully wrapped gift, and delightful card with a picture of a teddy bear. I opened the package and there, sitting in a little box, was a real teddy bear just like the picture, with a pink heart on a white knitted jumper saying 'I love you Mummy'.

Micheline asked me to take out the bear and pack him for our trip, and put him back in his box when we were safely home. So that evening, Teddy was packed in my backpack, ready for his round-the-world trip. It was going to be an exciting, yet tiring time for the little grey Teddy, and he would have his photo taken in many places around the world.

I made a lovely album for her sixteenth birthday, called 'Teddy's travels'. On the first page he is sitting shivering in the snow of New Zealand in late June 2001, and a few pages later he is sitting in Montana in the sunshine. Looking at the pictures now, they are a wonderful memory for me, as these views are no longer in my head. I turn each page, seeing each place, each event, each person. There I am holding Teddy, and there is a silver pen caption for each photo. I smile as I see myself in all the various places, holding Teddy, but there is a curious disconnection.

I cannot really recall being there, and have no other recollection around the event in the actual photo. It does not trigger any other sights or sounds to run in the video recall of my head. But obviously the evidence is before my eyes, so I was there and I can today still enjoy these past events by looking at the pictures, people smiling, interesting places, and some special family members that I recognise.

Teddy is there in each photo, and now he is over there in his box next to my desk, back from his travels. He is a reminder that he and I were really there!

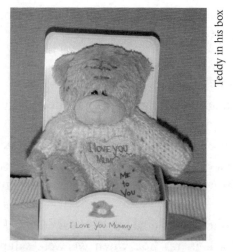

Teddy in his box

A whirlwind of media and packing

The weekend before our trip overseas, I was anxious, and felt as if I was stepping into the unknown. We were embarking on a global, yet uncertain mission to meet with others in Montana, and with ADI in London.

It was frantic, busy, packing, finding space for Teddy, deciding what to take, how many medications I would need, and so on. In-between this flurry of activity, we needed to remember to watch TV, to see some media coverage of our lives. That weekend, early on the Sunday morning, the programme Sunday Sunrise showed a segment called the 'Long Goodbye', about our lives together and our hopes for the future.

Most memorable for me was the shot of Paul and I walking hand in hand by the smooth lake in Canberra, on a crisp autumn day, looking at the black swans gliding smoothly through the water, as the sun just began to set. The colours were magnificent, and it was a very peaceful and meaningful moment captured on film. But in many ways it reinforced the image of walking into the sunset, rather than a new life in the slow lane, with new activities and opportunities.

However, another report, shown on the Monday, the 7.30 Report, gave a very different view, reporting that I had recently received my graduate diploma in pastoral counselling. The presenter opened our piece, saying:

> Seven years ago today, Christine Bryden was awarded the public service medal in the Queen's Birthday honours awards. At the time, she was a high-flying public servant, working in the Prime Minister's department. The following year, Christine was diagnosed with a form of dementia. ...she 'refused to treat dementia as an insurmountable barrier'.[14]

In my interview I said 'You can actually challenge that brain and rewire bits. I'm losing bits of brain, but I'm teaching other bits of brain how to do things.'

But perhaps I was overdoing it? Maybe I was doing a bit too much teaching of my brain? This trip to Montana and to London and back was certainly going to be exhausting, and maybe I should not step out like this, and maybe I should leave it to someone else to advocate for people with dementia? I know my daughters have thought that many times since my diagnosis.

I remember my eldest daughter Ianthe becoming quite exasperated with my busy and stressful life, saying to me, 'Mum, why can't you "do dementia" like any other normal person and just rest at home!' She was thinking, why did her Mum have to be such a 'workaholic', and keep on making such a huge effort, and getting stressed and tired because she was clearly struggling with a terminal illness. She was worried I would decline faster because of my strenuous efforts.

I can't answer that question she posed, as to why I have been so driven to change attitudes, to challenge the stereotype, except to say that I feel deeply for all those with dementia who simply cannot draw together the threads of enough energy, nor enough collected and collective thinking, and who are subjected to a great deal of misunderstanding.

Until you can truly try to see the world from our perspective, the people living this journey from diagnosis through to death with dementia, you cannot empathise, you cannot provide the care we need to travel this traumatic road. I simply hope that one day all people with dementia will be treated with dignity and respect, and our care partners and care workers will do all they can to understand our needs despite a lack of verbal communication.

It was this hope that took me to Montana.

Montana mountains

It was late June, and we walked down the slate steps of the airport arrival hall, past large moose heads and bear heads hanging on the walls. There was Morris Friedell, smiling, ready to welcome us to Montana. We chatted as he drove us to Laura Smith's family farmhouse, which was in a green valley, with mountains in the distance.

DASN had arranged over the Internet to meet at Laura's place, and a few mobile homes from around the USA were parked on the grass, and the house was bustling with arrivals. Lynn Jackson had already flown in from Canada, and Jeannie Lee from Hawaii. Jan Phillips and Mary Lockhart were both there, with their husbands, having driven from their US homes in their mobile homes. Carole Mulliken, Alice Young, and Candy Harrison were all there – it was a very joyful time to be meeting with people I had only seen as names at the bottom of emails, very special people to me who were sharing my journey with dementia. It was exciting to realise that all eleven of us were each able to communicate, to share, and to work together to try to achieve change as a group.

We agreed to meet together the next day, and Paul said he would help take notes. We talked about our chat room, our email community, and our vision of being a global internet-based advocacy and support network for people diagnosed with dementia.

Each of us had been through the trauma of diagnosis, and each one was searching for support and acknowledgement from our Alzheimer's Associations. Morris was full of praise for the Australian Alzheimer's Association, and how earlier that year in Canberra, it had been so receptive of the sessions for people with dementia, and was taking our views into account.

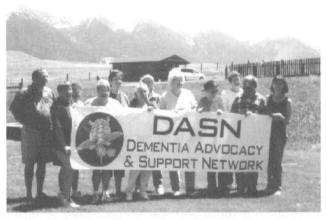

DASN friends in Montana, from left: Phil, Candy, Carole, Lynn, Jeanne, Laura, Alice, Mary, Morris and me

Paul carefully took notes, and each time we stopped for a rest, he would scurry away to Morris' room and type up a record, print it out and distribute it. But each time we resumed a topic, at least one of us had lost our notes, or forgotten to bring them along. We laughed, and realised we were coping despite our memory loss, and that we needed to acknowledge we were in a new area of endeavour, working together as people with dementia as advocates for the future. We could have a long and rational discussion, followed by carefully argued and agreed decisions, but we would all forget what we had talked about, and even lose the pieces of paper on which these agreements were recorded for posterity.

It was a true God-send to have Paul there to capture our thoughts, to reflect them back to us, and to patiently copy yet again our papers for us when we lost them. We agreed to call ourselves DASNI, adding international to the title, and volunteered for various tasks on the new Board of Directors. This new Board then met again after more rest time, to look at a proposal that Morris and I had drafted in the previous months.

The proposal to ADI

We had been emailing each other, developing this proposal for Alzheimer's Disease International (ADI), responding to its annual report of that year, which stated that: 'all the ordinary pleasures of life…are no longer possible' for the person with dementia, and 'The mind is absent and the body is left as an empty shell.'

We started the draft DASNI paper with the following paragraphs:

> The dominant paradigm for Alzheimer's Associations around the world to date has been the provision of support for care-partners of people with Alzheimer's Disease. Therefore by default the focus of Alzheimer's Disease International (ADI) has become the provision of care for people in the moderate to late stages of the diseases that cause dementia, and more particularly support for the families and care-partners of those with Alzheimer's Disease in the later stages.
>
> Now that diagnosis is occurring earlier, and anti-dementia drugs are available to retain function for longer, people with early stage dementia are themselves also seeking information, advice and support from local Alzheimer's Associations. However, current strategies are aimed at the later stages of care, and directed towards the care-partner, who needs a great deal of support in providing the type of care people with later stage dementia require.

Then we noted the new charter of principles being drafted by ADI, and how these contrasted with that bald statement about the mind being absent and the body remaining as an empty shell. We said that this type of thinking strips us of both respect and dignity, as clearly we are not seen as functioning, useful people.

The paper went on to talk about a growing group of people with dementia who want to rebuild their lives and to regain self-esteem, and need recognition and inclusion, opportunities to network and contribute. It finished with the following recommendation:

> ADI and its member organisations should make provision for people with dementia, as well as their care-partners, to contribute to the range of its activities including policy, program, conferences and advocacy and to participate in management and advisory structures.[15]

We talked about this paper as a group, sitting on a variety of chairs and cushions in the farmhouse at Montana. We agreed that I would take it to the head office of ADI in London the next week. Paul busily finalised the document and emailed it to ADI, making arrangements for us to visit while we were staying with my mum in London.

Looking back it was a momentous time. We adopted the slogan 'act locally, think globally' and we were excited at the prospect of trying to change the world, starting with that one small step of our meeting in Montana.

The farmhouse 'incident'

That evening, six of us went into the nearby town for dinner, exhausted but exhilarated with our newfound global advocacy action. Paul was the only one without dementia, but you would not have known it, to look at this motley, yet normal-looking group going into the restaurant. We studied the menus, carefully made our various selections, and then the orders started to arrive.

The waitress said, 'Who ordered the pasta?', and was met by blank looks, then, 'Who ordered the fish': more blank looks. And so on. Paul came to the rescue, allocating the right order to the right person. Thank goodness he was there!

A few minutes later, just as I was chatting to Lynn animatedly about our day's activities, I got stuck in mid sentence, as so often happens to me, as I tried desperately to find the word for the place where we had been meeting. Lynn knew I was trying to come up with the word 'farmhouse', and was about to tell me, but she was also struggling to hang onto the thought that we should order some wine, and so we needed to ask for the wine list.

At that very moment, as these two thoughts were tumbling about in her head, the waitress walked by our table, so Lynn caught her attention and said, quite firmly and clearly, 'Do you have a farmhouse?' meaning, of course 'Do you have a wine list?' But this is not what came out and not what the waitress heard. But the waitress took this in her stride, and started to tell Lynn that her family indeed did have a farmhouse, but that now they lived closer to town to help out in the restaurant.

As she went away, we all looked at each other and laughed. This was so typical of what could happen to us, as people with dementia – thoughts tangled up in our heads, crossed wires misfiring, and odd words coming out. Paul eventually caught the attention of the waitress and asked for the wine list.

We have no idea what the waitress thought of us – not knowing what we had ordered, asking about farmhouses, and yet looking so normal. Perhaps we should have stuck labels on ourselves that we were people with dementia, then maybe she would have understood. Or would she? Maybe then she would expect us not to be able to speak, or even be in a restaurant?

Going to London

The next day we were farewelling our new friends, my colleagues on this journey with dementia, and boarded the plane that would eventually take us via Toronto to London.

We found our way under the bridges and walkways of the busy rumbling of Waterloo station, to the insignificant front door of ADI. We buzzed and were let in, making our way up several flights of stairs to the offices. We were welcomed and shown into the small meeting room. Paul and I sat on one side of the big table. On the other side were the Chairman, Executive Director and staff officer of ADI. It was 29 June 2001, and what I have before me now are a few notes Paul took of that meeting.

The Chairman, Dr Nori Graham, outlined how ADI had been set up in 1984, and that it provided material for members, with the annual conference being its main activity. She was business-like, and quite formal, as she took us through the history and outline of current activities.

Then it was over to me to speak to the paper we had sent across from Montana. I felt as if I was being very carefully observed. Had I really helped to write the draft of this paper? Was there really a group called DASNI who had discussed it and submitted it to ADI? Or was Paul really the instigator, the person pulling all the strings? Was I some kind of ventriloquist's dummy?

I began by talking about DASNI and then outlined the proposal we had prepared, and its recommendations that ADI be inclusive of all dementias, and that it should provide support to people with dementia as well as their care-partners. We were also proposing that ADI and its member organisations should enable people with dementia, as well as their care-partners, to contribute to the range of its activities including policy, program, conferences and advocacy, and to participate in management and advisory structures. I concluded by saying

> We people with dementia recognise the tremendous support provided by ADI and its member organisations to our care-partners, and want this to continue. We seek recognition and inclusion alongside our care-partners, as companions on a journey of care.
>
> It's all very new territory, as we people with dementia are speaking out, maybe getting diagnosed earlier with the new technology, and given a new lease of life by the new anti-dementia drugs now available. We are using our remaining abilities to push the boundaries and to enjoy life while we still can. Thank you for giving me this opportunity

to speak to you on behalf of the Dementia Advocacy and
Support Network. I would be very interested to hear your
reactions to what we are proposing.

I finished talking and there was a silence for a while, then smiles broke
out all around, and Nori came over and said 'Is that a Maggie?', refer-
ring to my multi-coloured Australian designer jacket. We chatted
much less formally now, and it very quickly became clear to me that
this was a very welcome approach by DASNI, and that ADI was very
open to hearing our message of people with dementia wanting to be
heard, seeking to be included.

Within a few days, our new DASNI President, Phil Hardt, received
a letter from the Executive Director of ADI, thanking him for the
proposal, which would be circulated to all members in advance of the
international conference in Christchurch in October 2001. The plan
was to set up a working group to prepare a response for consideration
at the annual conference in Barcelona, in October 2002.

Phil replied, saying

> Your plan of introducing our recommendations to ADI in
> such a timely manner is to be applauded and your encourag-
> ing remarks to all members of ADI to begin including
> person's with dementia in meaningful positions is also enthu-
> siastically supported by DASNI. Such inclusion will make
> ADI the role model and benchmark for the future![16]

DASNI had made a difference! Our gathering, our working together
to stand in solidarity as people with dementia, had an impact, and each
one of us felt encouraged. We could almost hear the effect of our coop-
eration in 'thinking globally', and I see now what Hakuin, the Japanese
monk and famous writer, meant when he said 'If someone claps his
hand a sound arises. Listen to the sound of the single hand!'[17]

From such small beginnings in the autumn colours of Canberra, to
a gathering in Montana of people with dementia willing to think
globally, came this great step towards new hope for support and recognition for people with dementia. And it had all just taken three
months!

Christchurch – a chance to shine!

It was 'full steam ahead' for dementia self advocacy from that moment on. We got back to Australia, to the wintry chill of Canberra in late July, and there was an invitation waiting for me to speak at the opening plenary of the ADI conference in Christchurch, New Zealand, in October.

A wonderful lady, Verna Schofield, from New Zealand got in touch. She was on the ADI Board, and was a real champion of people with dementia. She helped make sure that at that conference in Christchurch there were sessions for us, and a quiet room; that we were involved in all sessions, and our voice was being heard.

There were quite a few from North America who decided not to come, given the changed world they now faced after 11 September 2001, but a few brave souls made the trip, including our newfound friends from Montana, Morris, Lynn, and Jan and her husband. It was so good to meet with them again, to celebrate what was being achieved since Montana.

The DASNI booth

Jan Phillips had put together an amazing booth to showcase what DASNI was, and what we stood for. The booth was a major attraction, as many delegates had not spoken to a person with dementia before, despite being active in the Alzheimer's movement. The DASNI logo was prominent in her display – a turtle with wings, and a 'forget-me-not' flower in its mouth. The slow-moving turtle symbolised our journey with dementia, the wings expressed our desire to rise above this battle, and the flower was there to remind you to remember us. The Nyanja of Malawi have a wonderful saying that captures how we felt, as turtles who had been able to fly: 'Little by little the tortoise arrived at the Indian Ocean.'[18]

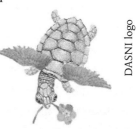

DASNI logo

Jan had prepared a basketful of bookmarks, with colourful ribbons spilling over, and brochures about DASNI. She had spent months at her printer, and buying materials, gluing and folding. There were ear plugs for us to use and to hand out, to help with the noise of the conference. There was even a video of each of us being interviewed during our time in Montana.

The results were spectacular, and Jan had created a masterpiece. Christchurch was truly a chance to shine, to launch our self-advocacy as people with dementia onto the world scene, setting in motion a whirlwind of change!

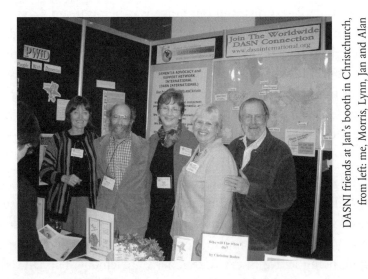

DASNI friends at Jan's booth in Christchurch, from left: me, Morris, Lynn, Jan and Alan

Challenging a stereotyped view

I was nervous, and shivering – not just from the cold of Christchurch – when we walked into the venue for the welcome session for presenters and other notables in ADI. This reception was being held the evening before my talk, when I was still incognito, an 'undercover' person with dementia.

I was sipping my wine and nibbling on a biscuit, when this very tall man and his wife came over to introduce themselves to us. He asked how I came to be involved in the Alzheimer's movement – this is a common enough question at such functions. But my answer was far from what he had expected: 'I have dementia, that is how I have become interested and involved.' He was speechless, and said he had never met anyone with dementia before. After this uncomfortable moment, we chatted and were soon able to overcome the awkwardness of my 'coming out' with dementia, and the challenge this presented to 'normal' expectations of what I should be like. I have become used to this type of 'introductory moment' now, when I have to say I have dementia, and deal with the reaction.

The next morning I gave the opening plenary address in the Christchurch conference centre, the first person with dementia to do so at the annual ADI conference. My talk was called 'Diagnosis, drugs and determination', about my journey with diagnosis, and how the anti-dementia drugs and a positive attitude had been important in maintaining function. I had prepared a new PowerPoint presentation, in rich pinks and purples, with striking pictures from computer clipart on each slide. I had also managed to insert my latest scan on one of the slides, to 'prove' my credibility as a person with dementia.

It was a huge hall, with over a thousand people there, and I was awestruck to receive a standing ovation. The biggest joy, though, was to be able to mingle with all my friends with dementia afterwards, and to feel not alone in being able to talk, in being able to present myself as something other than someone in the last stages of dementia. But I really needed all of their support. Someone overheard, after my presentation, a doctor challenging the scan that I had shown, saying it could not be mine otherwise I would be unable to talk. Was he saying I was falsely claiming to have dementia? Was he saying that I had put my own name on the scan, instead of someone else's? Yet again, I was not meeting the stereotype of someone in the late stages, and yet again I was facing a lack of credibility.

But here in Christchurch, there were others who were able to express how they felt and were challenging the stereotype. Jan had prepared an amazing booth, Morris had prepared an inspiring workshop (which was standing room only), and Lynn had given media interviews as President of DASNI.

This time I was not alone!

Meeting together

It was great to meet with over a dozen men and women with dementia, aged between 51 and 76, at special discussion sessions which Morris and I had prepared. We had a range of diseases (Alzheimer's Disease, vascular dementia, fronto-temporal dementia and frontal lobe dementia), and had been diagnosed from as early as 1990 to as late as the previous year (2000). We had come from New Zealand, Australia, Canada and the USA, and it was just so wonderful to share our feelings.

We talked about how our emotions – at times overwhelming and frightening – seemed to be out of control, and that it was like being on an emotional and unpredictable 'roller-coaster', which was embarrassing.

As we sat around in a group, it was really encouraging to realise that all of us felt that the spiritual dimension was important, whether this was religious rituals, the garden, music or whatever gave us a sense of meaning. We had a great discussion about animals, because they needed and loved you unconditionally, even if you could not remember their names!

Brian McNaughton from New Zealand captured the special nature of our group sessions so well and so poignantly in his letter posted to DASNI after the conference, saying

> We cried with each other as we told our stories and shared the fears of a progressive illness that would finally take our minds away, and laughed at the burnt toast, the half cooked dinners, the forgotten appointments and all the many wonderful situations only we with dementia get ourselves into.
>
> The love and support we received from each other created a passion that empowered mind and spirit. This gathering was a most rewarding and encouraging experience. We shared laughter and tears, deep dissertations on living and dying. Through it all we gained strength from being together. It humbled me greatly to experience the depths of faith and humanity and the heights of love and support offered by my fellow journeymen.[19]

Handing on the relay baton

For DASNI, the ADI conference in Christchurch in 2001 was a wonderful affirmation of those tentative steps taken in Montana earlier that year, of local action translating in global outcomes. And it was a real boost to receive a letter from the ADI conference organisers:

> You created a world first for people with dementia actively participating in an ADI conference – and in doing so, added a unique glow to the conference. Your example has achieved a great deal by creating a precedent that will encourage others to follow.
>
> In being so open to talking to other conference participants and to the media, and the DASNI international stand, awareness of dementia has been considerably heightened in this country. Public misconceptions have also started changing about the effects of early stage dementia and the capability of people to manage their everyday lives. This was a precious gift to offer.[20]

DASNI had indeed offered a 'gift' to ADI and to the global dementia movement, but in many ways for us people with dementia, it was a relay baton that we had handed over, not a gift. It was only the beginning, the first steps.

We felt like we had been the first runners in a relay race. We knew we could only run the first stretch, because each of us had progressive illnesses that would take our ability away bit by bit, so that we would no longer have as much energy to try to change attitudes.

So we ran this first part of the race, and we handed the relay baton over to ADI. From then on, ADI was off and running the rest of the race.

Barcelona and beyond

Soon after the Christchurch conference, another ADI working group was set up, and it included three people from DASNI, as well as a person with dementia from the UK, Peter Ashley. The previous ADI working group (leading up to that conference) had been looking at ways to include people with dementia in the life of ADI, but this group was to be more task-focused, revising the ADI Charter for Principles of Care and developing a fact sheet for Alzheimer associations and the ADI intranet pages.

DASNI was looking forward to the next conference in Barcelona, in October 2002, and again Phil wrote to ADI proposing that a person with dementia be invited to present a plenary address on the first day of the Conference, that there be special sessions for people with dementia in a quiet room, and a booth for DASNI.

Lynn and I met once more in Barcelona, but Jan and Morris had been unable to make it, and our other Australian and New Zealand friends were not able to come, so we were a much smaller group. But Jeannie was able to come over, all the way from Hawaii, and it was great to see her again, a year after having first met her in Montana.

We unpacked the box for our booth, and took out some great T-shirts and caps that Jeannie had prepared for DASNI, as well as unloaded the brochures we had printed in Australia. As we were busily arranging and sorting all the materials, an English gentleman came over to introduce himself. It was Peter Ashley, who we had 'met' over the internet as part of the ADI working group, and who was going to give the plenary address the next day.

We were thrilled to sit in the audience and see Peter give that speech in Barcelona. The chair of the session was overcome as he finished, and we all stood up clapping. A very small group of us, people with dementia from Australia, Canada and the USA, were in the dark of that audience, cheering our colleague as loudly as we could, encouraged that someone from the UK was joining in our efforts in advocacy.

But by early 2003, some of us in DASNI were flagging, tired, no longer as focused or determined, less able to self-advocate as actively as before. We were also perhaps a little disappointed that the Barcelona conference had not been able to support the attendance of more than just a few of us. And we were each just a bit further into our individual journeys with dementia.

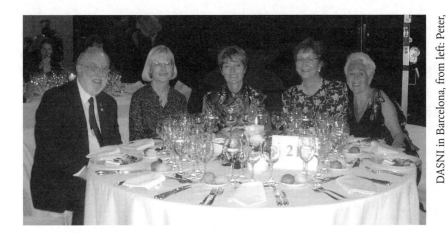

DASNI in Barcelona, from left: Peter, Marilyn, me, Lynn and Jeanne

But we had handed the relay baton onto ADI, and Verna Schofield was setting a furious pace. At times I was unable to keep up, and felt discouraged and dispirited at the inevitable conflicts that occurred, but she was a great encourager, writing to me, saying, 'You know, you are a constant source of inspiration to me. Whenever I start to flag, I think about all that you have achieved in the past few years and the truly remarkable pace of change made in promoting the cause of people with dementia since the last Alzheimer's Australia conference.'[21]

> You talk…about passing on the baton. The image that arises for me of your advocacy over the past couple of years is of a stick being carried down a fast flowing stream, with you and DASNI members providing the momentum of the rushing water. The task of others was helping to keep the stick flowing freely until it reached calmer, more accepting waters.[22]

Looking at her words, they help me see the big picture whenever I feel like giving up because of difficulties in the short term. I realise I am floating on a fast stream, carried by all the supporters of people with dementia around the world. It is truly exciting to see so much happening so quickly!

But we were all exhausted by mid 2003. It had been a long two years of struggling to keep afloat on this stream, yet we felt relieved that others would benefit – those who would follow that journey of a devastating dementia diagnosis, and then a feeling of exclusion both from society and from those organisations supposedly set up to assist families with dementia. Perhaps from now on, the person living with the diagnosis would find the help they needed.

For those of us who had met at the farmhouse in Montana, it had been a long two years of battling with our losses and our decline. Yet a few of us remained active in cyberspace to see the fruit of our labours – to see how acting locally and thinking globally can actually change things.

And we were amazed by the speed at which the international movement was working. The last part of the relay race was gaining momentum, and little did I know that I was to be expected to continue running in the race, to keep hold of the baton. It all became evident at the next ADI conference in Santo Domingo in 2003, which was to bring with it a huge surprise!

Whatever next!

Paul and I sat in the back row, watching the ADI Council members as they worked through their agenda. There were at least 50 countries represented around the table, and it was awe-inspiring to see the global dementia movement at work, collegiately and supportively working to improve the lives of families living with dementia. And people with dementia from Scotland, Canada, Puerto Rico and Australia were there, joining them at the table.

It was hot and sticky in the Dominican Republic, and we had walked for half an hour to get to the hotel where the meetings were. We were on the other side of town, in more modest accommodation, along with South American countries, India and Pakistan. I was a bit sweaty from the walk, and very confused from finding our way across town, and then gaining access to the room for the meeting.

I was having difficulties walking along unfamiliar streets, and Paul had steadied me by holding my hand so that I would not stumble and fall. I found the traffic, and the sights and sounds of our walk challenging and disturbing for my thoughts. By the time we reached the venue, I was flustered and agitated, and it was difficult to settle into the meeting. So I fidgeted and looked around at the representatives from all the member countries, as we sat down in the cool air-conditioned room.

I had reluctantly agreed to be nominated for a possible seat on ADI's Executive Committee, as ADI had decided to have up to two people with dementia on this committee. This was a great outcome from the working group recommendations, but I was hoping others would be able to take up this opportunity, so giving me more time to rest and be with family. I was feeling 'burnt-out' and tired of running this race, advocating for people with dementia.

So I had mixed feelings about the nomination. I was not sure of the procedures, nor what was going to happen. All I knew was that voting would be later on in the day, so I was relaxed and simply watching what was going on. Orien Reid Nix, the Vice President of ADI, stood up to report on the outcomes of deliberations on governance. As she gave her lively and visionary presentation, we heard about the new campaign for World Alzheimer's Day, 'No time to lose', encouraging all members to unite their efforts in raising awareness about the global impact of dementia. DASNI was mentioned several times as a valuable network of people with dementia throughout the world which can provide input to ADI activities, both through local and national associations, as well as directly through the Executive Committee.

By the time Orien had finished speaking, I began to realise that people with dementia had been nominated alongside others, for the two vacant positions on the committee. Should I be one of those elected, I would have equal responsibility and accountability for a period of three years. This was an alarming thought for someone with a progressive illness! I had hardly recovered from this realisation, it seemed, before the votes for the five nominees were being counted, and there I was elected to the board of ADI for three years!

I stood up, my heart in my throat, as I said, 'I feel humbled and honoured to be elected, and will do my best to represent the 18 million people around the world who are struggling, along with their families, with the various diseases which cause dementia.'

I still feel every bit as overwhelmed as I did that day, to be trusted with the honour of this task. Mind you, part of why I felt so overcome with the thought of further work and effort was the sheer exhaustion I was experiencing by the time of the Santo Domingo conference. You see, this was just part of a round-the-world trip to talk at various conferences and seminars, trying to help improve dementia care.

Round the world in 80 days

It truly felt as if we had gone around the world in 80 days, like the old movie! But rather than travelling by hot air balloon, we had flown on a number of airlines in a special ticketing arrangement. Paul had managed to organise a trip which included India, Israel, France, London, South Africa, Brazil, Santo Domingo, Taiwan and Japan. It had only taken just over 70 days, but it felt like I had been away for ever!

It had all started in Barcelona in 2002, when quite a few people from a number of ADI member countries expressed interest in my giving a talk about an insider's perspective of dementia during 2003, timed to coincide with possible travel to the 19th ADI conference in Santo Domingo.

Thankfully, before Paul sold his motorbike to pay for this huge trip, we received generous support from two pharmaceutical companies, which market the anti-dementia drug Aricept which keeps me well enough to continue advocacy.

Our first stop on the journey was Cochin, India, where we had a delightful visit to the day care centre. One man there who now has Alzheimer's used to be a top bureaucrat. He was regularly given a file for his complaints, which were duly attended to and returned to him on file. He was still the 'boss' despite his dementia! The former station master had his afternoon tea at a small table in a room very similar to his workplace, so also was made to feel very comfortable. I was impressed by this person-centred care.

My talk was on the major local holiday of Onam, yet there was a large crowd in the heat of the afternoon, including an impressive array of consultants who supported the local Alzheimer's Association. Amongst the audience were many nuns, carefully dressed in pale blue and white habits, sitting demurely and quietly, very attentive to my speech. At the end, the chairman stood up and gave a very emotional response, quoting from Rudyard Kipling's poem 'If', using no notes, just his excellent memory. There were quite a few moist eyes, including mine, after he had finished speaking!

Next stop was Goa, India, and a welcome from the very capable team at the local Alzheimer's Association. They had organised for the press to attend the meal at the venue where I was to give a short talk that evening, and this resulted in front page media coverage, including a cartoon! I was amazed, and could not imagine how dementia, or me, could in any way feature on a cartoon.

The next day we were driven to the venue for my main talk, where I unsteadily climbed quite a few flights of stone stairs with Paul's help. In the room, a computer was being set up for the PowerPoint presentation, and people gathered to take their seats. I was introduced to two people with dementia and their families, and I was again impressed to see the caring way in which they had been included.

The next stop on this trip was France, where I had been invited by a charitable foundation to give a talk and meet with French Health Ministry officials, to promote awareness of dementia and the need for better care. I found that an important issue was the stigma surrounding dementia, and in particular attached to the French word 'demense'. An example of this seemed to be the fact that a person with dementia from DASNI had been invited to attend – all expenses paid – but his family were reluctant for him to come.

In a short introduction in halting and very bad French, I mentioned the recent heat wave, of the hot summer of 2003, and the consequent deaths. I raised the questions: how many of those who died might have had undiagnosed dementia? How many of them might have forgotten to drink enough water?

Paul talked with health officials about the fact that in many ways Australia and France, like other Organisation for Economic Co-operation and Development (OECD) countries, are very similar, with an aging population, and a time bomb ticking of a future dementia epidemic. As the 'baby boomers' age, diseases that cause dementia will become more common, and they will impact very greatly on an under resourced health care system.

We travelled then under the Channel by train to London, and soon seemed to reach Waterloo station. The ADI head office was just nearby, and we trundled our baggage through the tunnels and along the street, back to the small upstairs meeting room where we had met with ADI only two years before. We had a cup of tea and a chat before facing the London Underground to rest for a few days with my mother.

I really needed to 'recharge my batteries', to rest and recuperate, for the next part of our trip. We were off to Israel, and I was scared, anxious and apprehensive. Travel warnings had been issued by our government and we had been advised to defer all non-essential travel. But Paul felt it was important to take the message of dementia care to our friends in Israel.

I gave a talk at the conference in Tel Aviv, which was attended by almost twice as many people as had been expected. The audience was talkative and active, people walking in and out, talking and moving about, mobile phones ringing and doors banging. I found this all very distracting, and the chairwoman asked that the doors be closed and asked for quiet so that I could continue. I managed to get through my talk, and my overheads behind me on the screen had been translated into Hebrew. I went outside to rest, feeling so tired from the effort of trying to focus with this background visual and aural distraction.

One highlight for me from the conference was talking in the sunny courtyard during the break out time, to the person who had just given a presentation on service dogs for Alzheimer's patients. These dogs will return you home when you get lost or when your care partner feels you should return home, and will also recognise signs of distress and activate an alarm button. I felt this was a wonderful idea, as companion pets are such forgiving care partners, who do not mind you cannot remember, or find your way, or even know their name!

As we travelled back in the bus from Tel Aviv to Jerusalem, a young woman who had emigrated from the USA to Israel was chatting with us. Just before she got off the bus at her stop, she asked if, later in the week, I would be able to give the same talk at the dementia care centre where she worked. The staff had been looking for a speaker to give them a spiritual boost, as they were feeling depressed and very down-hearted at the situation in Israel. I agreed, but felt exhausted at the thought of another talk.

A few days later, we were driven across the picturesque streets of the Jerusalem landscape, with its stone buildings and barren rocky hills, to an area just outside of the 'green line'. On our arrival at the centre, I was led to a quiet room, with a soft calm feeling about it. Just outside was a herb garden to sniff and flowers to see. This time of quiet gave me a rest, to gather my energy for the talk.

In my talk I talked of 'dancing with dementia'. This phrase I use to describe how Paul and I are a care-partnership, adapting my care as I journey into areas of different need. I referred to Psalm 30 from the Bible: 'You have changed my sadness into a joyful dance; you have taken away my sorrow.' The women reached into the pockets of their long skirts to bring out their well-worn psalm books.

We shared the words of this psalm and of others, as I talked about the role of my faith in overcoming the trials of dementia. The lady who had invited me was delighted, and said it was just what they needed. I was honoured that I, as a Christian, could give spiritual comfort to my Jewish brothers and sisters.

From Israel we travelled to South Africa, where we were greatly honoured to be introduced to a man who had been active in the uprising. He took us around the main sights of Soweto, the birthplace of this new nation. We then travelled several hours south to Bloemfontein, where I gave a talk to the national conference, and managed a few words in Afrikaans. My mother is from Belgium, so I speak some Flemish and have a limited understanding of written Afri-kaans. Our delightful hostess had helped me to find a poem by Ingrid

Jonker which was used by Nelson Mandela in his State of the Nation Address.[23] I selected an appropriate part, about a child being at all meetings, looking through the windows, into mothers' hearts, and becoming a man, yet lacking a pass. I opened my talk with this extract – of course with a very Flemish pronunciation!

I asked the audience to think of this child, this man, as the person with dementia, the one who is often forgotten as a human being, who is looking through the windows of our meetings about dementia, and is often excluded. I spoke about how we are all part of a rich tapestry of humanity, saying, 'Truly we must include all people with dementia when we say 'ubuntu' – we are together in our great humanity... Like Mandela we people with dementia can transform a personal tragedy into a triumph. We need no longer be the forgotten ones who have forgotten how to remember.'

As I sat down, the chairwoman was too overcome to speak at first, and hugged me tightly as she gathered her composure. At this conference, I was particularly impressed by an African psychiatrist, who spoke with passion and vision. The challenge seems to be to gain information about dementia in the African population.

It was indeed proving to be a 'whistle-stop' tour, and from South Africa we flew on to Brazil, where we were going to meet for the first time another friend from DASNI, who is a supporter of people with dementia, and runs a day care centre and a monthly carers support group. We let her know that our ticketing arrangements took us through Brazil, and she was so excited! She arranged a medical symposium in Belo Horizonte, and it was a full day of excellent presentations, with my talk translated by her, page by page. All the attendees seemed to be delighted with the outcome of this spontaneously arranged event.

For Paul, this visit was extra special, as he had once lived for two years in Brazil and was keen to show me Rio and Belo. So we managed some brief sight-seeing in-between our talk commitments. All too soon we were off once more in an airplane, this time up across the vast continent of South America, and I was thrilled to see the huge Amazon snaking below.

We arrived in the dark warmth of a Santo Domingo night, and I was anxious about how we were going to get to the hotel, as this would be the first place where we had no arrangement to be met by friends in the dementia movement. But as we made our way out of the inevitable passport queues, my name was called out and there was a member of staff from the pharmaceutical company which had sponsored us, ready to take us to the hotel!

The ADI conference in Santo Domingo marked the end of the race in my exhausted eyes, after this trip and all that had gone before. The relay baton had reached the finish line, and people with dementia now had a voice which would be listened to, in order to improve the way people with dementia are included and supported in the global dementia movement. I was astounded by what had happened since DASNI's modest start as the Coping With Personal Memory Loss email group in 2000, and the speed with which an international organisation such as ADI had responded to our advocacy.

But for me, there was still a little more of my own race to run. Our next stop after Santo Domingo was Taiwan, where we flew in to a memorable orange sunset. A member of staff from the company was there again to greet us, and she and our hostess had made such wonderful arrangements. We were shown into a suite in a top hotel, which was to be a haven of rest and peace in our journey, on this frantic rush around the world. I treasured this special time, and felt rested and at ease.

I gave two talks, one to a large hall full of carers and the other to a small meeting room of medical specialists. It was a busy three days, and we ate some delicious Chinese food. Yet again the question of my diagnosis was raised. I still find it hard to comprehend why this should be so. Why would I lie about this? Why would I not get this diagnosis checked and re-checked to be sure?

From Taiwan we flew across to Japan, and as we taxied in I saw a camera crew out on the tarmac. I said, 'Paul, I am sure that crew is filming our landing, and will be there when we get out of the queues.' He was not convinced, and said surely it would be for something else.

But as the doors to the arrival hall opened, there was the camera crew, alongside our dear friends who we had met just earlier in the year.

You see, I had met Noriko Ishibashi at the DASNI booth in Christchurch and she had videoed my talk, and bought my book despite not understanding a word of English. After her friend translated this material, she was so excited and set about getting in touch. Noriko has been inspiring, and energetic in her commitment to working to change the care environment for people with dementia.

She had brought a group of friends to visit us earlier in the year, and it had been a very special time, captured in an appendix to the Japanese version of my book, which had just been released as we touched down in Japan. Across culture and language, Noriko and I had been able to truly communicate at the deep level of spirit to spirit, and to share our thinking on how best to improve the care environment for people with dementia. And it was Noriko who had been instrumental in our visit for these ten days in Japan.

We boarded the bullet train, and sped smoothly above the city and around the bay, to our hotel and the venue for my first talk. From our very first moment in Japan, we were cared for by an attendant, there were quiet rooms at each venue, and each hotel was wonderful. I felt very special, treasured, taken care of, so that I could really relax and rest. Indeed my time in Japan was one of the most peaceful and enjoyable trips I have ever experienced, meeting such dear new and old friends who took such good care of me!

I was overcome by amazing generosity and attention to detail, and felt welcomed with enthusiasm and a shared sense of love for people with dementia. There were lovely flowers, thoughtful gifts, claps and smiles, and rapt silence and earnest questions for each talk. I felt very honoured and privileged to be given this opportunity to share.

I recall clearly a dinner after my talk in Okayama, when a wonderful young man who was devoting his life to care of people with dementia, said to me 'I used to think of people with dementia as being far away. But now, after hearing your talk, I feel they are close by and that I will be able to reach them.' This was such insightful thinking, and I was so impressed by this young man, who was young enough to be my son, who was able to express the centre of the message, the key to caring for people with dementia.

The highlight of the trip was in Matsue, where after my talk I was presented with a wedding kimono! I put it on and stood hand in hand on the podium with Paul. He was wearing a lovely corsage of flowers on his jacket that he had been given, and we stood smiling as the audience clapped and clapped. It was like getting married all over again! And the highlight of our trip was that night's stay in a Japanese inn in Matsue, overlooking the lake. I had stayed once in such an inn when at work, but now I could share this very special time with Paul.

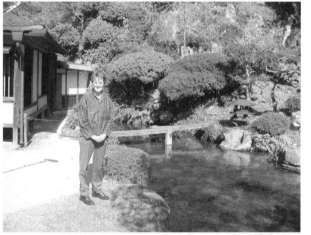

Tranquility in Japan

We then travelled to Kyoto, the venue for the ADI conference in 2004, and saw the beautiful conference hall high above the city with its temples and castles, alleyways and cobblestones. Our interview for NHK TV in a Kyoto temple was such an honour. It filled us with the sense of mystery and history, as we walked around the peaceful autumn colours of the gardens, and contemplated the majesty of nature in each leaf and tree.

A monk met with us for Japanese tea, and he talked with us of the importance of nature, and how the bud represents the whole potential of life, and how the simplicity of a carefully arranged garden reflects the divine. I shared how as a person with dementia, I live in this 'now', in the beauty of this natural environment, focused on the beauty of each flower and leaf. I talked of how as a Christian I focus on the joy of each day, of each moment of my life in God's beautiful creation. It was a very special time of sharing across faiths and cultures, and between a person with dementia and a wise master. We connected spirit to spirit and were able to exchange a deep sense of meaning.

At the nearby headquarters of the Japanese Alzheimer's Society, a large group of people were gathered around the huge conference table as we walked in, with our dear attendant close by. She was able to help us share my thoughts on what it really means to have dementia, and what remains as the core of the spirit within. We were greatly honoured to hear from the President and the Secretary-General of the Society. They were the driving force for the forthcoming ADI conference in Kyoto, and had clearly done an amazing job of organising this event.

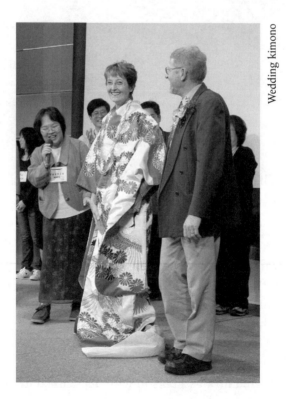

Wedding kimono

It was very special to know that the Secretary-General, a medical specialist, had shared a dinner table with many of us in DASNI at Christchurch in 2001. Now, so much had happened since then, and along with his colleagues in the dementia movement, he had been an important part of this move for change.

When we finally arrived home we heard that the national broadcaster NHK had produced two television programmes about our trip, and as we watched them on our video, it helped me to recall memories of this special time, our dear friends, and the beauty of Japan. I could in some way reconnect with the serenity that I had felt during this trip, where I was so well taken care of, and was able to share a real sense of meaning, intimacy and relationship across culture and despite language.

I really needed to rediscover this sense of peace that I had discovered during my time in Japan. I had felt a tranquillity that was like an emotionally serene island amidst the stress and anxiety that I was experiencing. Not only had we just got back after two and a half months of travelling in so many different countries, but we came back to settle into a new house!

I wouldn't recommend that you move...

Yes, we had ignored the medical advice and moved house, not once but twice in two years. I was feeling very agitated, very anxious and very stressed. I now realise why that advice was so wise. I need routine. I need the reassurance of knowing where I am, where things are, even if it is not easy to find them.

Our first move maybe was the result of my impulsiveness, as I was losing more of the control available in my brain. I simply had enough of the cold in Canberra, of the stress of giving talks and of media interest. This was in 2001, that frantic year of moving from local to global action. On our way to Montana, we visited my cousin on Bribie Island just north of Brisbane in mid winter. The Island was sunny and warm, and the sun glimmered over the peaceful water of Pumicestone passage. It seemed like paradise!

We visited again on our way to Christchurch, and by then I was determined to move. I insisted, nagged, argued, seeking a way out from the stress. I thought that by moving I could escape this stress. I did ask, though, our church minister, Neil, and my spiritual advisor, Liz MacKinlay, to come and pray with us about this decision. They both found time on a busy Christmas Eve in 2001, to sit in our kitchen and put my crazy idea to God. Just a few weeks later, another minister friend, Bill, was visiting. He came downstairs one morning, and said 'I have a verse for you, from the Bible, which says "You have gone around the mountains long enough, now is the time to head north".' Of course, Canberra is near the mountains, and Bribie Island was a great distance to the north.

Moving to Bribie Island in March 2003 was really counter-intuitive. It all seemed so fast, so amazing, so totally what a person with dementia could not do. When we visited my neurologist and told him what we were planning he said, 'Well, I wouldn't recommend that you move, but given that you have seemed to survive a trip around the world, maybe you will be able to cope with this.' Not exactly a ringing endorsement of our plans, but at least he was not going to stop me following my impulses.

And certainly our first year on the Island was less stressful, and there were fewer demands on my time. But I found it so hard to settle, to remember the new faces I was meeting each day, and I was so disconnected with all that had been familiar in Canberra. The landscape was so different, the air and light new and strange, and we were now 1500 km away from all the familiar faces of my friends and family.

I was struggling, and found it hard to cope with the stress of events in early 2003. There were terrible bush fires in Canberra, affecting each one of my daughters who lived around the area where we had once lived. It had been devastated by fire, 500 homes destroyed and countless lives traumatised. By May 2003 my middle daughter, Rhiannon, had moved back home and there was more change in my life.

I wrote to my friends in DASNI: 'I am struggling a lot now. My book was written in 96 and 97, and now I can't even start the second one I hoped to write. My thoughts are jumbled, and my apathy…just makes each day seem a muddle.'

The muddle became even more frantic and distressing, when we decided to move again, to an acreage nearby, so that we could share the adventure of developing a run-down, swampy piece of overgrown land into an exciting horse property. Again I think it was my impulsiveness that drove us, my temporary excitement, my moments of lucid thought, and my determination, that swept us along.

By early August 2003 we had moved, and plans were made for the fencing, clearing, re-seeding, drainage, stables and so on. Just three short weeks later we were off overseas for our long trip. We had not unpacked into our new house, and I had no home that I really felt was my own.

So when we arrived home after Japan in late 2003, I felt homeless. I did not know where anything was, and could not find a routine for dressing, showering or going to bed. Everything was strange and unusual. I stumbled and fell several times, and had a very sore hip for several months. My body was exhausted and my mind stretched beyond its meagre capacity.

It took me almost six months to start to recover some energy, and some feeling of a centering in my life again. And of course, I needed to find the energy to get to the computer and write this book, all about having dementia, living this life in the slow lane, and making a long journey of diagnosis and treatment, and of self discovery and reflection.

3

Let's Talk About Having Dementia

The medical journey

Diagnosis with Alzheimer's Disease

My journey into finding out all about dementia, from an insider's perspective, started with feelings of stress and of exhaustion, as well as the occurrence of frequent migraines.

The doctor finally sent me for a routine CT (computer-assisted tomography) scan in April 1995 to check that there was no brain tumour or lesion causing my migraines. The report said: 'The ventricular system, sulci and CSF [cerebrospinal fluid] spaces are more prominent than expected for the patient's age, indicating a degree of generalised cerebral and cerebellar atrophy.'

I talk in my first book of how I then had an MRI [magnetic resonance imaging] scan, which noted 'generalised enlargement of the ventricular system and subarachnoid spaces indicating generalised cerebral atrophy'. The first neurologist that I saw said the scan looked as if I had probable Alzheimer's Disease and that I should retire from work immediately. This was an enormous shock for me, so I saw

another neurologist in July 1995, who carried out more scans, an elec-
troencephalogram, and blood tests, including for AIDS (autoimmune
deficiency syndrome). I rested at home to recover from the migraines,
from my stress of trying to cope at work, and from the added trauma of
the possible diagnosis of Alzheimer's Disease.

By August 1995 I was well enough to do a complex battery of
exhausting psychometric tests, and the report noted 'difficulties in
attention/concentration, speed of information processing, and appli-
cation of strategies to more complex and novel verbal and visual
material, [which are] consistent with frontal lobe damage'. The report
noted the generalised cerebral atrophy visible on the scans, and said 'a
provisional diagnosis of early stage of Alzheimer's Disease seems the
most likely'.

The neurologist carefully reviewed this report, and ordered further
tests and scans to ensure that there was no other reason for the brain
damage and resulting loss of function. These tests included a lumbar
puncture to check for signs of infection, and a small bowel biopsy to
check for Whipple's disease.

He then informed my doctor that he had 'not identified a treatable
alternative diagnosis to early Alzheimer's Disease', and recommended
that I start taking the anti-dementia drug, Tacrine, 'to try to preserve
memory function'. He strongly recommended that I retire from work
as soon as possible. So in October 1995 I started taking Cognex
(Tacrine), and started to arrange for medical retirement from work.
Over the next few months, the fog started to lift from my brain, and I
managed to start to deal with the trauma of my diagnosis. I went back
for regular check-ups from 1995 to 1998 while on Cognex, which
confirmed continuing brain damage and yet a slowing functional
decline, perhaps due to the effect of this anti-dementia drug. I settled
into a new life with Alzheimer's and wrote my first book, working
through the emotional and spiritual journey that I was travelling.

Re-diagnosis with fronto-temporal dementia

In 1998, as discussed in the first chapter, I had further scans. The CT scan reported 'brain atrophy affecting mainly the frontal lobes'. I also had a PET (positron emission tomography) scan, which reported:

> There has been a definite but slight progression in the degree of cerebral glucose hypometabolism and also the degree of cerebral atrophy. The atrophy is most marked in the mid to superior frontal lobes and the interhemispheric fissure is much wider than 3 years ago. It is associated with more marked reduction in glucose metabolism in the mesial frontal cortex, particularly in the region of the cingulate gyrus… There is also hypometabolism of both temporal lobes with the suggestion of temporal lobe atrophy bilaterally. All the changes are more marked on the right. There is mild but definite progression since the study performed three years ago. The findings would be consistent with a fronto-temporal dementia rather than the pattern seen with dementia of the Alzheimer-type.

It's important to recall that PET scans look at function, which was increased due to my anti-dementia drug. I have seen scans of Alzheimer's brains with and without Tacrine after ten months, and the difference is very marked. Imagine what little function I might have shown on my PET scan, if I was not taking Tacrine. By 1998 I had been on Tacrine for three years!

I had further psychometric tests, which confirmed this finding and led to my re-diagnosis with fronto-temporal dementia, rather than a dementia of the Alzheimer type. In the three years, it was clear that the damage was more severe in the frontal lobes. The neurologist told me that some fronto-temporal dementias are Alzheimer's like, and stabilise for many years. This was very encouraging.

But this re-diagnosis meant little change in terms of treatment (for example, I was told to continue taking the anti-dementia drug), as fronto-temporal dementia has many of the same symptoms as Alzheimer's and other dementias. However, it is less characterised by memory problems, and more by initial personality changes and problems with speech and judgement. Indeed, fronto-temporal dementia is probably still very much under-diagnosed.

Mind you, remember how unique we each are – so different in the way we use our brain. So even two cases of Alzheimer's are not the same, let alone the other types of dementia. There may be considerable misdiagnosis of Alzheimer's Disease, particularly in those under 65 years of age, when checked out at autopsy. This diagnostic error is particularly true when simple behavioural tests are used and not followed up by scans and blood tests, as well as more sophisticated psychometric tests.

At the time of the reassessment in 1998, the neurologist said he thought the brain deterioration was now 'glacially slow', and that I had a lot longer to live than the five to ten years previously thought. He was not following statistics, which would estimate that I would deteriorate just as fast, if not faster, with this type of dementia. He was treating me as a unique individual.

Following up each year...

By February 2000, the neurologist wrote:

> [Christine is] being treated for a chronic fronto-temporal dementia. This is a slowly progressive cerebral degenerative disorder which has a slow rate of progression. She has significant difficulty with memory and with some executive functions, sufficient for her to require increasing levels of supportive care. Medication with Tacrine has a slight long-term beneficial effect but no other active treatment is available.

In May 2001 it was time for a follow up MRI scan, which reported:

> Cerebral atrophy is present and it is more focal in the frontal and temporal lobes with prominence of the silvian fissures. There is, however, also a degree of central atrophy and atrophy involving the occipital lobes. Cerebellar atrophy is

also present... Though the fronto-temporal atrophy is certainly more well established than atrophy elsewhere, it is present elsewhere including a degree of central atrophy.

The neurologist reassured me that although the pattern of fronto-temporal dementia was clearly evident, it appeared to be progressing slowly.

In early 2002, further psychometric tests showed selective deficits in memory, spatial location, executive function and speed of information processing. This simply supported the decline being seen in the brain scans, and the diagnosis of fronto-temporal dementia.

By November 2003, the MRI showed that

> There is prominence of the subarachnoid space over the superior cerebral surface, more prominent in the frontal that the parietal region. This extends into the para falcine region. The subarachnoid space is also widened in the middle cranial fossa of the anterior aspect of the temporal lobe... There are three small foci of high signal change in the periventricular white matter in the parietal lobes. This may reflect mild small vessel ischaemic change.

The radio nuclide brain perfusion study also showed further functional changes in the fronto-parietal cortex, compared to previous studies. So the damage to my brain still continues, slowly but surely, despite my apparent level of function.

What does all this mean? Well, basically that I have much more wasting away of the brain than expected for my age, and that this wasting away is steadily getting worse. Each year, more and more of my brain is disappearing. The bits that are going are in the front, and in-between the two big halves (like those of a walnut) of the brain.

When I give talks I usually put a scan up on the overhead, because often people just can't believe there is anything at all wrong with me. The pictures clearly show atrophy (wasting away of the brain) in the frontal and temporal lobes, which is apparently (according to my neurologist) even more marked in the computer read-outs than the scans.

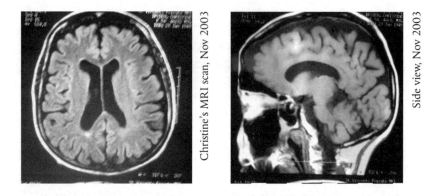

Christine's MRI scan, Nov 2003

Side view, Nov 2003

Sometimes I also show another person's scan, with no brain damage, and the 'pictures are worth a thousand words'! Usually there's a sort of hushed silence, as people who know what brains should look like try to take in the fact that here, right in front of them, is someone who should not be able to do what she is doing – that is, give a talk!

According to the doctors, my scans are like those of someone in the moderate stage of fronto-temporal dementia, ready to be admitted to a nursing home. It's like a 115-year-old brain trying to power a 55-year-old! But my functioning is as if I am only in the early stages. Why is that? Why can I function with so little brain? Why can I still speak, dress myself, write this book, read, study counselling, and so on?

What does this mean to me? Well, that a normal person exists behind the scans and diagnoses, and this particular person who has a dementia has no intention of going quietly or declining as expected by much of the medical profession – but fortunately not by my neurologist, who is happy to talk to me each year, speaking to me as if I still have a brain and deserve to be treated as a normal intellectually functioning human being.

He gives me hope by not assuming anything, by not giving me any projections of decline, and by basically saying that I am and will be as good as I feel and that there is still much to learn from patients such as myself and everyone with dementia.

His explanation of why I seem to function beyond the expectations from my scans is that I had a much higher level of pre-existing capability on which I seem to be drawing now. He says 'She is managing as well as she is partly because of the unusual very slow progression of her illness and because of the excellent support of her husband.'

Paul and I are dancing with dementia as best we can, but he was not there at the beginning of this journey. He joined it only after the first three years of struggle.

A journey through trauma towards hope

The struggle began with the testing for the initial diagnosis. It was an agony of waiting, wondering and desperately hoping that whatever is wrong can be treated and life can go back to normal. My life changed dramatically when I faced the shock of diagnosis. It feels like a curse when the doctor says, 'You have dementia. There is no cure.' It's like the pointing-bone of a traditional curse, and what is said often leads to a terrible depression. For me, I certainly withdrew for a year or so, writing my first book, processing my thoughts and feelings.

Many of us have heard at diagnosis what we now refer to as the standard dementia script: 'You have about five years till you become demented, then you'll probably die about three years later.' No wonder we often suffer depression and despair! Dementia and Alzheimer's are both words that create fear and dread. Many of us wish we had cancer. At least then usually there is talk of treatment, of chemotherapy, of possible remission. There is none of that with a diagnosis of dementia.

What do you tell us at this critical time of diagnosis? 'It's best not to let her know.' 'He doesn't really understand.' 'Go home and enjoy the rest of your life.' The assumption is that nothing can be done, so why bother? But we want to get our life in order, to think about family relationships, our legal and financial affairs. Give us information about dementia. Don't assume we lack insight, for we might simply be in denial – a perfectly normal response to the shock of diagnosis.

One really frightening thing for you when you are diagnosed with a dementia is that no one knows how fast you might deteriorate – it is hard to get across how that feels, each day you wonder what faculty might be lost. You don't know if you'll be able to read and write, or add up for much longer. Setting up an enduring power of attorney might reassure you about your financial affairs, but it reinforces this fear of losing 'the three Rs' (Reading, wRiting and aRithmetic) and of how shameful that will be. And what about the loss of giving up going out to restaurants, concerts, the cinema, the club, golf or church – largely through shame and lack of understanding?

For the first two years after diagnosis, I tried desperately to believe that the damage had always been there. The brain damage is stark. Maybe I had been born with that amount of brain missing and coped very well despite it? Or maybe what I had could be cured? But now I realise I do have a progressive dementia, and importantly that there is treatment and hope. I have learned to live positively with dementia, and my neurologist has done a great deal to help me by treating me as an individual who can still achieve things in life despite dementia.

For example, he wrote in late 2003:

> There has been a gradual progression of her cognitive disorder, but she has managed to fit in a sponsored lecture tour on the problems of being affected by dementia... She has the most interesting combination of excellent insight and reasoning skill despite declining short term memory and language abilities... It is fairly clear that Christine's dementing illness will continue to evolve at the same rate as it has in the last eight years, so that there is no need to consider any major changes in her life activities.

My neurologist is a continuing source of encouragement to me, and treats me as a person first and foremost, not a disease. He gives me hope that I can function to my full potential despite my decline.

But my potential is not what it was before I became ill. My friend Margaret, who used to work with me, was being interviewed by Yuji Kawamura of NHK, the Japanese national TV network, and said that I 'was just so quick to grasp anything that was put before her. Any problem was not a problem once it got to Christine, there were always solutions to any problems that were presented to her.' I am no longer that 'brilliant' person she describes, but there is more to me that I am discovering as I journey inward with dementia. Again, as Margaret said 'having this dementia brought out all the compassionate side of her…she became a much softer personality.'

My functioning seems almost normal because of my anti-dementia drugs, without which I could not travel, talk or even shower or dress. But not only these help, but also my previous level of education and ability. The neurologist says it is like I used to juggle maybe as many as six balls whereas ordinary people might juggle three at most. I might have dropped three balls now at this stage in my decline, but I still juggle almost as many balls as the ordinary person I meet each day. I treasure some delightful juggling balls that were given to me in Japan, after having mentioned this analogy in one of my talks there. They remind me of how I once was, and how I am now, and inspire me to keep juggling as best I can!

Hopefully I have enough extra time, and insight, to share with you what it feels like to struggle with these diseases that cause dementia.

What it feels like to live with dementia

There is such a terrible stigma attached to this disease that no one wants to talk about it or admit to a diagnosis, even seek one. So we struggle to remain 'normal' and pretend we are feeling fine. But we are not – it feels very different now to how we once felt. We know what it felt like to be normal, and that is not what it feels like now. And as the disease progresses, it becomes more difficult to describe how we feel, to get our thoughts in order and actually get the words out so you can understand us.

The first signs of dementia are very gradual changes in ourselves, so that we hardly notice it. Our family and friends might think 'we are not ourselves', and we might think we are just stressed. But it is the beginning of a long slow journey of change.

I felt foggy in my head and became more readily confused. I was very tired, and just wanted to come home from work and sleep. But I couldn't give up and go to bed. I was a single mother with three girls to look after at home, as well as up to 30 staff and a budget of several million Australian dollars to worry about at work.

I was so stressed out by ordinary things and was getting terrible migraines every week. I would forget things in mid sentence, get confused about finding my way to work, and found it increasingly difficult to make decisions. Everything was an effort and something felt very wrong!

The psychometric tests were exhausting and I was puzzled as to why some things had seemed so hard and yet others quite easy. I had great difficulty remembering numbers, making pictures into a story, working out what was so special about arrangements of blocks set out before me, and making my way through a maze. My mind was often blank when trying to recall the various shopping lists and stories.

We face a daily struggle to cope. Each day is filled with a myriad of activities which become more and more difficult as time goes by. Each task seems bigger and more overwhelming, so that we lose the interconnectedness of our thread of life. Life has become a fragmented kaleidoscope of problems as we juggle an enormous pile of difficult tasks.

We feel as if we are hanging onto a high cliff, above a lurking black hole. Daily tasks are complex. Nothing is automatic anymore. Everything is as if we are first learning. Cooking burns, ironing is forgotten, washing is no longer sorted, and driving becomes scary. You tell us that we have asked you that question before, but we have no recollection. It is just a blank for the past, and this feels strange and scary, and yet you are frustrated with us.

If we had an arm or leg missing, you would congratulate us on our efforts. But you cannot see how much of our brain is missing and how hard it is to cope, so you don't understand our struggles. For me it's like struggling to live in a fog, especially without Aricept. Everything is confusing, and the struggle is exhausting to the point of extreme tiredness.

We ebb and flow like a parallel universe of untreated and treated dementia. We have our good days and our bad days. As my friend Morris from DASNI said, there are 'windows of clarity' which we must take advantage of. But unpredictably we can feel exhausted, confused, muddle-headed. Life seems too difficult and we retreat.

Laura, the pioneer of DASNI, captured our feelings so poignantly in an email she wrote in early 2001, as part of a study into early onset dementia:

> Most of the time I live in the space I can see and the time called 'now'... It is almost a 'virtual world'... I move...and a new space opens to view...like a new room in a computer game... There is a type of cheese, I forget its name, that when thinly sliced is very lacey... my life feels like that – so full of spaces that it barely holds together...or like a tree in a gusty wind...branches touch and connections are made but fleetingly...made and unmade, little sense of cohesiveness...even my rooted-ness to my place in space feels tenuous...as if I might be torn loose, uprooted, blown away.[24]

You see, it is far more than simply memory loss. We are confused, we have problems with our sight, with our balance, with numbers and with direction. It is a real disease, not a normal part of aging. We have no sense of time passing, so we live in the present reality, with no past and no future. We put all of our energy into *now*, not then or later. Sometimes this causes a lot of anxiety because we worry about the past or the future because we cannot 'feel' that it exists.

But this fact that we live in the present, with a depth of spirit and some tangled emotions, rather than cognition, means you can connect with us at a deep level through touch, eye contact, smiles.

> Your talk has helped me so much to understand what my mother is going through. She could never really tell me, and I always feel so helpless. Now I know much more about how it must feel for her. Thank you for giving so much of yourself to us this morning.

THE LADY SPOKE to me, tears welling in her eyes, expressing the emotion, the pain, of the years of not knowing, and now of the awakening, the feeling that she at last could have some more insight into her mother's view of the world, what her day was like, what her journey had been like for her as she declined into Alzheimer's Disease.

I had just finished yet another talk, organised by my local Alzheimer's Association, for family and professional carers. I felt wrung out, after a 45-minute talk followed by questions, but the honesty of this lady's openness, her struggles expressed wordlessly through her tears, meant it was all worthwhile.

I have given many talks over the past few years, in Australia and overseas, to professional workers and family care partners, to dementia training courses, and at conferences and each time the response is the same. The talk – even though to me it sounds to be just the same thing, modified a little, over and over again – has been a real insight into the world of the person with dementia, into our struggles each day to cope as our brain disappears.

At one of my early talks, an exciting thing happened. A fellow stood up in the audience and motioned to his wife to speak out for him. She said, 'We came to your talk last year, and we're here again. He says that he found what you said really described how he felt, and your suggestion of ear plugs for noisy places has really helped.'

This was the first direct confirmation I had that what I was saying, others felt too. That was until I joined my email support group, and found that 50–60 of us around the world felt that way too. As Jan said in one of her messages 'You continue to astound me. I am in awe of your ability to organize and communicate so clearly "our" needs. I have printed this out and shared it with my husband.' And Mary Lockhart, likewise, said 'Just the way I feel also. I am so glad to have you on our team.'[25]

But I feel as if time is running out. I visited Canberra recently, where we had lived until a few years ago, and it was a very special time of reflection for me. I felt very relaxed and happy, and found that the beauty of the natural environment, the plants and the landscape forms, were strong visual memories which somehow restored my spirit. The beautiful gum trees, the possums, the parrots and the crisp cool air gave me a very spiritual time, and I felt a great peace filling me. Yuji, from NHK, was talking with me one morning about all these feelings.

I struggled to talk, as tears welled up in my eyes, because beneath this sense of peace was the awful feeling that I don't have much time left. It is such a struggle to get my thoughts and ideas out. Yet I feel like a sputtering candle, as it dies down to the last few centimetres of wax, the flame flickers just a bit more brightly before it finally disappears.

I want so desperately to get all my ideas across, and I am doing my best with this book, my last effort to put them all down on paper. I am anxious as I seem to be less and less able to capture and communicate these thoughts. There is a stream of ideas coming through my brain, yet they don't remain there. They are fleeting glimpses of insight, there one moment, totally gone the next. Unless I speak them out, or write them down, immediately, they are lost forever.

I feel that God is giving me all these ideas, but maybe I didn't write them down fast enough, maybe I have waited too long to write them all down. But it's a horrible feeling to be like a dying candle, burning bright at times, but running out of time, because I feel there is much to do and I have responsibilities for my daughters.

I try in this book to share how it feels, so that you can help us as we journey further into our decline with these diseases that cause dementia. I have tried to structure this section so that it more or less follows our journey of decline, both from our perspective, and from the point of view of what you can do to help us.

I am doing all I can to communicate what it is like to have dementia, but it is becoming increasingly difficult. People often say, 'Oh, you're doing really well! You look so well.' But I am very scrambled in my head.

Each day, life is such a struggle!

I described my feelings to a reporter recently:

> I am more stretched out somehow, more linear, more step-by-step in my thoughts. I have lost that vibrancy, the buzz of interconnectedness, the excitement and focus I once had. I have lost the passion, the drive that once characterized

me. I'm like a slow-motion version of my old self – not physically, but mentally.[26]

I'm like the swan, gliding above, paddling frantically beneath. My functioning seems OK at the surface, but just below, there are my legs paddling frantically to keep me afloat. And it feels as if I am paddling faster and faster each day. It seems as if I'm going to sink soon, because the struggle is getting to the point where I feel too exhausted to keep going like this.

When I talk to the neurologist and tell him what I am doing, he sees the swan, and yet underneath, when he examines the tests and scans, he can see how fast my legs are going. I can still swim a bit and put on a good show, so that you don't notice much is wrong. Nobody knows, except me and my poor damaged brain, how bad it is. It would be a lot easier just to give up, because it is a struggle everyday.

Effort and exhaustion…

These characterise our day. It tires you out just pottering about the house, making a huge effort to remember what today is, and what is happening today, and what you plan to do today. No one really understands how hard it is to live life like this, so everyone seems to trivialise how we feel, patronise us, and make out they feel the same way. But we know that's not true, because we get exhausted by just the very simple things each day. And we also know what it felt like to be normal, to have 'normal' difficulties, which people claim are just like ours.

I am no longer a 'can do' person. Often I just can't do something – it is all becoming so hard to struggle to cope each day with this damage in my brain. The complexity of so many things is a source of anguish. Just getting up, how to make a cup of tea, how to go and have the shower, where are my clothes and what shall I wear. I can't decide what to wear. Many decisions are simply so complex and I can't remember what has been said or offered so can't decide. It is much easier to 'go with the flow'.

Cooking is so complex and almost beyond me now. I have to line things up along the counter in order of the recipe, then use them, then put them back so I do not use them twice, and have to write down each step of the timing. I become exhausted, taking all day to do this, making notes, making sure everything is there, planning, laying the table, then trying so hard to make sure I remember to serve each part of the meal. Washing, sorting, deciding – life is full of struggles and complexities.

I suppose the anguish is because everybody doesn't seem to know how difficult it really is, that every moment of the day is a conscious effort to do something, whatever it is. What is normal in this abnormal disease? We can be tempted to maintain a cheerful facade, and deny anything is wrong. You may either go along with this and deny dementia, or assume we lack insight and take over our lives.

We cannot win. If we pretend at normalcy, increasing energy is required to maintain the self, so less is available for you, and for coping with stress. We may show a catastrophic reaction to what may seem to you to be a simple challenge.

If you take over our lives, then it is so easy for us to withdraw into helplessness. Life is so hard anyway, and you can make it so much easier for us. But in so doing, because we need constant repeating of actions and thoughts to keep remembering, we will lose functions daily. It would of course be easier to give up and withdraw, and be helped in every way. I wouldn't have to struggle. But then I fear I would lose so much function, as each day I have to try harder to remember what skills I still have.

Even walking and seeing are hard...

Stumbling, wobbling and spilling are features of daily life. I find I cannot walk along unfamiliar ground without looking down at my feet, and going up or down stairs requires careful attention to each step and each action. My vision and the signals that my eyes send to my brain to interpret are slow. In turn, the messages that my brain sends to my body to respond to what the eyes see are also slow.

The result is that the world feels like a wobbly place, and it is hard to know where each part of me is in space. My environment around me swims in and out of focus, as my head moves and my body walks. And my body is slow to react to the changing environment. I had some bad falls a few months ago, walking in the paddocks, and my friends in DASNI often talk of the falls they have had. Now Paul holds my hand to steady me.

When I am holding a glass of liquid, it is a huge effort to try to keep it from spilling. I have to look at the glass, look at my body, take care of how my body is placed in space – there are innumerable actions and reactions in this seemingly simple task. For me, carrying a drink has become a major challenge. Where is each part of me in space? Where is that glass and why does it slosh over unless I stare at it? Why does it bang into objects suddenly in its path when I lift it across the table? How come when I reach out, I knock over things and make a big stain?

It's like being blindfolded, looking through a tunnel. My peripheral vision seems to be more limited and I startle at or keep getting distracted by apparent movement around me. It is as if I have blinkers on. If I walk past a mirror, I can be startled by the strange person in the room with me!

I often knock things over in the kitchen or bathroom. I misjudge distance and bump into things. Patterns can confuse me, so I may stumble if walking across a smooth yet patterned floor. It just seems as if all I can see is in front of me, and someone has blindfolded me so I cannot see what is alongside me or around me.

Very slow reaction time

The world goes too fast and I am too slow. As a passenger I am a driver's worst nightmare, as I assume you have my slow reaction times and get very stressed out at the speed you are going, how close you are to the car in front and how quickly things are happening around us. So I startle, shriek, tense up, make comments! Paul's middle name is patience when it comes to driving me anywhere! And I get exhausted by city traffic, so much so that we carry an airline mask to cover my eyes. This helps a great deal, especially at night, when all the lights and movement are much too fast for me.

If you still drive when you have dementia, you wonder how long you will retain this independence, and are fearful of a minor prang as this will mean everyone will assume it was because of your dementia. Giving up your licence is a major trauma for the person with dementia and family. I only drive in emergencies now, and am very anxious when I am just going a few streets from our house in the quiet of our rural district. I feel I really cannot react fast enough to anything unexpected, and find it very hard to focus and to concentrate on the road ahead, as well as remember all the pedals and levers and dials and lights, which way do they go, what do they do, what must I do next.

Unreliable memory

Memory comes and goes, so that there are glimpses of past events, or future tasks I wish to do. But I can't find the memories when I want to, they only appear unpredictably, and I rush to note them down or to tell Paul so he can remember for me. It feels as if I will forget everything that is not written down.

The black hole of life unremembered...

I had once made a long list of things I wanted to remember to do, and was looking for it one day. Paul said he didn't know it was so important, and just thought it was a piece of paper and threw it away. I was so upset, so distressed. The horror of losing that list hit me – it felt as if I had no future. A black hole opened up behind me, and in front of me.

I screamed and shouted 'I don't know what I'm doing, this is terrible.' It was a real calamity, a crisis. It felt as if my life had been thrown away! Paul realised that there was no way I would calm down, that I was really suffering a catastrophic stress reaction. So he thought about where the list might be, and ended up going through the garbage bin, in the road, because it was garbage night. He emptied all the garbage, and found it.

I was very, very happy. So that's when we started to put a 'to do list' into the computer and kept on updating it. Now it is just a few short notes in the diary. For everyone else, this is just a list, but for me, this is my life. This is the only way that there is organisation in my life. Otherwise it's just a complete mess, because inside my head is a complete mess. And every now and then a thought comes in, and I think, ohhh, I must write it down. That thought won't pop into my head again on any sort of reliable basis, it is like a spinning wheel of words and phrases, randomly coming to rest.

Intermittent reception and fog...

The unreliability of my memory is as if the printer ink is running low and it sometimes works and sometimes doesn't. Some days I can remember this morning, but on other days I can't. It is such a hit and miss approach to a life gone by. Your memory is erratic. Sometimes it feels as if a black curtain has fallen over what has just gone by. You are in a continual present, but through that curtain is a vivid past that existed some years ago. Yesterday or today, last week or the week before, are a blank. Just writing in a diary might be a help, but then we have to remember to find the diary, and to look at the right page!

It feels as if there is cotton wool in my head, a sort of fog over my thoughts and feelings. This fog means it is hard to focus, to pay attention, and to keep up with what is going on around me. It leads to intermittent reception of life as it passes by.

I do not have enough energy to cope in the fog to find thoughts and get an idea or to work out what you are saying. Study, prayer, ordered thought and quiet reflection are no longer are possible. It is just a muddle of random thoughts. I go with the flow and make the most of the random bursts of energy and lucidity.

Conversations are full of questions and are a source of stress, as I am much slower and cannot respond quickly. I have lost immediacy. A simple question like 'Where is Paul today?' and my mind goes blank. I find it hard to understand what people say to me if I miss a few words and can no longer make sense of it. The missed word makes the sentence full of conflicting, meaningless sounds. And sometimes even if I hear everything you say, it sounds meaningless, just a jumble of sound and I need to ask you to repeat it again.

Have I asked you this before?

This intermittent reception applies to what we have just asked you, too, so we will ask the same question again without any awareness we have asked before. And we need to ask you questions to address our anxiety about an issue.

Paul and I, for example, went to a wedding of some dear friends at our church one Saturday morning. That afternoon, Paul said, wasn't it lovely this morning?' I said 'What was?' I had no recollection of what surely was a major event in that particular day. But the curtains had fallen across behind me.

Yes, it does drive you crazy to hear the same thing over and over, but how much worse is it for the person with dementia who knows they have asked you a question, but can't remember your answer? I often ask a question, and realise by the expression on the person's face that I have asked this before, maybe even only a short while ago. Sometimes one of my daughters will say, in frustration, 'I told you that before!' But I have no memory of the answer, so need to ask again. Please be patient with us.

One of my frequent questions is 'Have I seen this before?' for a book, a movie or TV show. And even if the answer is 'yes', I still find the storyline new and captivating. I have no memory of what happened before. But reading a book or following a story on TV is a struggle, as I cannot recognise the faces or names, nor remember the plot as it unfolds.

Where is it – you took it!

I put things in the wrong place. This is because I am walking around with something, going to put it somewhere, then something else pops into my head and I put that thing down, and of course cannot recall later where that was.

I have not hidden things on purpose. And I can't remember where I've put them. I can't even remember that I had it in my hand, so I am just as likely to accuse you of taking it and hiding it.

That's a very typical day. I do the tidying up and of course, that's useless isn't it, because to the question 'Where did you put it?', the answer is obviously 'I don't know'.

I need lots of clues

Some things I register and then forget – so if I am reminded, I might have some recollection. It is no longer under my control, and I need you to prompt me with lots of clues. It's as if I have lost all but one remaining key to the filing cabinet of my memories. You can help me try to retrieve a memory by finding a word, or a sentence, or a description of the event. I remember trying to describe this feeling to Paul when we were in the hotel in Kyoto. I pointed to the outline of squares on the paper shoji screen behind us. I said 'Each of these boxes is like one of my memories, kept locked up behind a little door. This is a wall of doors, a whole screen full of them, but I can no longer see behind this screen.'

I need you to find keys to these boxes, with a word or a phrase, to unlock the treasures of memory that have been locked away. My keys are lost, and I have this two dimensional feeling, of a blank wall of memory doors behind me for which I have lost the keys. Give us clues so we can join in with your memory and do not be upset if the key no longer fits the lock, or the store of memories behind the door has faded. Often I simply stay blank and have no recall to share.

Questions like 'Do you remember?' will make me panic. The black curtain falls down behind me as I desperately try to search for some recollection connecting to what you are asking. My speed of information processing is far too slow. Descriptions of your own recollections are much more helpful, as these give me time to think and may also sometimes these trigger my memory so I can share my own feelings with you.

But other times I do not register the experience, so even if I am reminded, I have no idea of it ever having happened. But I'll pretend it did. Paul can tell from my vague look, and the way I slowly say, 'Oh,…right.'

I can't really remember writing my first book, except that it took a long time and was difficult. But writing it, talking it through with Liz MacKinlay, helped to build up my sense of self, and to reflect on my personhood.

Not knowing labels

A name without a context is a real challenge. One day, Rachel, my daughter's partner, took me with her to look at plants when we were visiting Canberra, where we used to live. She said, 'We'll go to Phillip first, then we'll…' My mind fogged up, puzzled and perplexed. What was this thing called 'Phillip'? A person, place, shop, building? Only when we got to our destination did I realise that this was the name of our familiar shopping suburb. Rachel and I had a wonderful day, as I rediscovered in my head somehow a few of the real places that belonged to disconnected labels of my old home town.

I am slowly learning how to live without remembering labels: your name, or even my name. I know faces and know I connect with them somehow, but not why I know them and what I know about them. It is a world in which I know that I know you, but not why I know you.

Your name, the label that belongs to you, often is not there. Your face is familiar somehow, but meeting you happens too quickly for me to search through my disjointed memory and find a label for you, or a context of why I know you, or any information that might belong to what I know about you. I need time and clues, not questions. Try to chat about our shared experiences, so that I can find out why I know you, then maybe your label will appear. Don't just give me your label, as I need more than that to really know who you are. I need some detail as to why I know someone of that label.

When we visited Canberra recently, and saw my friends at church and at the Alzheimer's Association, I realised something quite important about the way I recognise people. I would see a face, and know it well, and there would be a spark of recognition, and of joy in knowing. I would then smile and hug these dear people. I knew they loved me for who I am, and was therefore confident to say to them, 'It's really lovely to see you, but I can't remember your label, I can't remember your name and who you are.'

You see, I did not know their name, whether they were married or not, whether they had children, if they had a job. I knew nothing about them, nothing in the 'normal' sense of how you know people and recognise them. The way I know people is in a spiritual and emotional way. There's a knowing of who a person really is right at their core. But I have no idea who they are, in terms of who they are meant to be in your world, of cognition and action, and labels and achievements.

This 'knowing' at the level of spirit, of a significant other, exists without the need for labels formed by cognition or even emotion. But I wonder if there would be a block to my knowing you, if you were upset that I did not know your label, your name, and who you are and why you are important to me?

Is my 'knowing' you triggered in some way by a connection with you, a response from you that reaches spirit to spirit? If you are hurting because of my lack of cognition, will this prevent me from knowing you? I do not know this yet, and of course, if and when it happens I will not be able to tell you.

I usually enjoy each moment of our time together, so why is it so important that I remember it? Please keep visiting me, even if I might not remember that you came before, or even who you are. The emotion of your visit, the friendly feelings you give to me, are far more important. It is the emotion I connect to, not the cognitive awareness of the event.

Why does it matter if I cannot remember, if I repeat myself, or forget what you told me. If I enjoy your visit, why must I remember it? Why must I remember who you are? Is this just to satisfy your own need for identity? Your visit is not a cognitive experience that I will store and recall. Let me live in the present. If I forget a pleasant memory, it does not mean it was not important for me.

I connect at the deeper level of spirituality, so I treasure your visit as a 'now' experience in which I have connected spirit to spirit. I need you to affirm my identity and walk alongside me. I may not be able to affirm you, to remember who you are or whether you visited me. But you have brought spiritual connection to me, you have allowed the divine to work through you. This can happen across cultures and languages, and is a very meaningful depth of communication, one that perhaps we should all strive for.

Anxiety and distress

What behavioural and personality changes are associated with my dementia? Certainly I have problems with speech, and maybe I do get more teary than before. Yes, and also maybe I am more demanding, less certain and more impulsive, and less in control than before. But hardly the sort of thing I had read about – of outbursts of anger, of becoming someone so very different to whom you were before. If anything, friends say I am nicer than before. But my family see me in a panic, out of control, unable to cope.

When I asked Ianthe, she said, 'Well, Mum, you used to be so focused' and Rhiannon said, 'You say "I can't do it!" now. You never said that before, you were always a "can-do" person.' But although my behaviour might have changed, I still feel very much me. I am here in the world around me, as long as I take my anti-dementia drug. Without it, I withdraw and retreat to my own small world. Everything is too busy and confusing.

On the edge of panic

My stress tolerance is very low, and even a minor disruption can cause a catastrophic reaction, where I shout or scream, panic and pace. I need calm, no surprises, no sudden changes. Anxiety is an undercurrent in our disease. I feel I have to do something but can't remember what. Often it feels like something terrible is going to happen, but I have forgotten what it is. With the stress of many activities at once, I become very focused, trying with all the brain I have left to concentrate. Telling me to rest won't help, but helping me to complete the task will.

Panic attacks come upon us like storms, expressing an inner conflict as we desperately try to cope with stress. We sense imminent doom. Please help us and give us a break from the effort of coping. If I am overwhelmed by stress, my brain reacts to this struggle with a migraine. Another way for us to deal with stress is apathy – to switch off, because of overload. There is simply too much happening at once to bother to try to cope. It's not a lack of interest, but of energy.

Anxiety is not something we can control – that controlling bit of our brain is missing. So we are reliant on you to help us calm down – but telling us to not worry is not the way! We have no resources to do that. Creativity is what you will need! What would you do with a troubled toddler – divert attention, help complete a task and give reassurance.

We have reason to be anxious. For many of us not being able to write and read is a real worry. Getting dressed or undressed is a stress, as we try to work out what to wear and how to put it on. And of course we know we cannot remember things, so are always worried we will lose something unless we keep track of it all the time. We fret as we cannot remember what we are supposed to do – is it Monday, morning or afternoon, was there something I promised to do, was there something I planned to do, is there washing to hang out or bring in, did I agree to ring someone? All these thoughts spin around and get us nowhere as we simply cannot remember.

Maybe in some way we are not stressed if we cannot remember? But that is not how it is for me at the moment. One day perhaps I can become used to not being in control, not knowing about what I am supposed to do, and to relax into my dementia, as it were, then I could be without stress. Perhaps this is what I have to look forward to as I progress with this illness?

But now quite often I have this feeling that I have forgotten something that I should have remembered, and it is important that I remember it, but I can't think what it is because obviously I can't remember. And it might be something terrible is going to happen if I don't remember it, and it just goes on and on like that.

Any unfinished job preys on my mind, nagging away. I might forget this task if I do not do it right now! So I persist at the task to the point of exhaustion, and get fatigued. Then I become irritated, blank, pacing around, not able to start or stop anything. I can't break the task into manageable bits, so I just keep on going, hoping it will become clear as I proceed.

I worry constantly about finances, about the future, about our bills, about what has to be done, what is on my job list. I feel so out of control that I can't cope with any uncertainty. I have a rising sense of frustration, much closer to the surface now, so much so that I can understand how someone without words might hit out physically when they have lost the word for 'no', when someone is trying to make them do something they don't want to do. I want you to make sure I want something before you force it on me. I am grown up now, and may not want to listen to your music, or play your games or eat what you want me to. I am worthy of dignity and respect, even if I cannot speak.

Constant reassurance is needed so that anxiety does not turn into a catastrophic reaction. We are all individuals, there is no 'right' way of doing things. Families must remember who this person was before their diagnosis and help the person to maintain as much independence as the person with dementia is comfortable with.

Pacing and wandering

I often get very distracted and agitated, for no apparent reason, but it seems to arise mainly from this undercurrent of lack of recall and possible forgetting of something important. So I pace around almost like a caged lion, or simply can't sit still, particularly in the evening. Often my cat will come to me and look anxious too, so I offer my lap to her, and she comforts me with her warmth and purr. My cat is a pure-bred Oriental, so is very focused on her owner, much in tune with my mood and needs, and always needing to know where I am. She is my dementia cat!

I find it difficult to settle at night, probably because it is hard to follow the story on TV, the adverts are noisy and disturbing, and even reading is tiring and difficult. If I retreat to a warm bed and into a routine of sitting with my cat and a book, this helps. Also, I take half a tablet of Oxepam at night, which calms me, takes away the feeling of a knot in my stomach and tension in my neck and shoulders.

I do get into a complete mania on occasion, at any time of the day, when I become focused on a task. I cannot be switched off nor jollied out of it. I become exhausted but oblivious to anyone's efforts to reassure me and divert me. Paul then simply quietly helps me by working at the task with me, reassuring me in some way that it will be done. As my neurologist commented, when I told him this, 'Paul is more valuable than drugs.'

Pacing around somehow releases the tension, the movement distracts me from the real issue of not knowing what day it is, what time it is, and what I am meant to do. I can't think what I am meant to do, but walking around makes it feel as if I am doing something, and releasing that pent-up energy inside of me, that frustration with not knowing what I am meant to be doing.

Background noise or vision...

These make it worse by scrambling the brain. Background noises and motion – like at shopping centres, doctor's surgeries, and often dementia day care centres and nursing homes – with radio, TV, telephones, people talking – make it exhausting for me to keep following the thread of what is happening, and I become very tired. Is this noise and motion at these places because the staff are bored?

The noise or motion feels like an egg beater in my head, scrambling what is in there and putting a static sound or visual screen over what is coming in. It is as if I have lost the filter in my brain, to focus on one thing out of many. Sounds can become a 'hubbub' and I can't make out what people are saying to me. Sometimes it is difficult to recognise sounds. If the doorbell and phone ring at the same time my mind freezes, unable to work out what the sound is or what to do. It's as if the sound, so loud, has blanked out my brain.

But if the music forms a pattern, it can soothe me and become a gentle part of the background. It needs to be regular and harmonic like Baroque, or familiar and soothing like Mozart or Enya, to settle me down, as long as I am not expected to do much at the same time. If the music is challenging, loud and not familiar, then I become anxious, scrambled in the head, and unable to listen, speak or think. All I hear is whatever sound is loudest and this bangs around inside my head, bruising my brain, grating against any thoughts or words that are there.

My functioning is as if I am walking a tightrope – I cope very well while I am well rested and not under any stress or any conflicting demands. But if the phone rings as well as the doorbell, or two people ask me a question at once, or I am tired or stressed, then I become confused, unable to think what to do, and my mind simply goes blank.

Tiredness of the brain...

After any mental activity, say at the computer, reading or having a long conversation where I need to concentrate and pay attention, I get very tired. I feel somehow 'scoured out' inside my head. My tiredness is of my brain, not my body, so that I simply need 'brain time out' – sitting quietly alone, with no noise or activity around me. I could still go for a long walk, maybe with someone to guide me who says very little, so my brain can rest.

When my brain becomes overloaded and fatigued, it's like a short circuit, and my brain cuts out. I get a blank, brain-less look and withdraw from what is around me. I'm not really there, my eyes cannot focus, and I can't say much. The fog thickens and I can't follow what is being said or is happening around me. Speaking, hearing, walking: all then become difficult after overload, and I need routine and familiarity within which to cope and to regain my sense of self.

I have heard that dementia disturbs the circadian rhythm of our bodies. For me, it feels as if I have permanent 'jet lag'. I toss and turn waiting for sleep, and it is as if I have lost the 'off' switch in my brain. I find that visualising calm places in my mind, or praying, as I wait for sleep, is increasingly difficult. I can no longer hold onto images or words in my head. It all becomes a muddle of emotions bubbling up from what has happened through the day, so increasing my distress.

My body is tired, muscles relaxed. My thoughts are not unpleasant
– no worries or anxieties. But my brain simply will not switch off and
let me go to sleep. But less sleep makes the anxiety and confusion
worse, so I use Temazepam to help me sleep. Warm milk, a warm bath
or relaxing music can also help.

Either I can't get started or I can't stop!

I had a wonderful email 'conversation' with Lynn, the President of
DASNI, who also has been diagnosed with fronto-temporal dementia.
She said, 'I am finding that apathy some days can play a really big part
and I do not feel like doing anything. Do you find that too?'[27] And I
replied, 'Yes – it feels as if everything is too complicated, too difficult,
and I can't decide what to do so I drift around.'

Our 'conversation' continued as I said, 'You cannot imagine how
much I can relate to what you are saying!!! On my good days it is like I
have a bundle of energy and can race around (in the morning only
usually), and get a lot done. I get very manic, wanting to finish everything *right now*, and don't know when to stop! I rush around till I get a
headache, and usually am exhausted by the afternoon, and by the
evening all I can do is sit and wait for bedtime!' Lynn replied, 'This is
exactly me. I have been plagued by headaches in the last while…I
never was a person to get headaches but now I get them frequently.'

An example of how focused I can become was when I wanted to
clean our house at midnight, it could not wait till tomorrow, it had to
be done right then. There was no way I could sleep. So Paul got out the
vacuum cleaner and patiently helped me clean the whole house.
Finally we sank into bed at about 2 a.m., and I was happy, yet distressed that clearly I was no longer in control of these urges and
impulses.

I flare up, say bad things, decide to move, to travel, to give away
cats, to adopt cats…my life seems to be a continuing drama of new
things, when I should be trying to stick to a routine.

And you cannot imagine what it is like to go shopping with Lynn
and me! Well, Paul is a most patient man, and waited for hours as Lynn

and I tried to make up our minds at countless shops. I find that any choice is just too hard. Do I want tea or coffee? – even this is a hard question for me. How can I possibly hold onto the information of all the alternative possibilities in a clothes shop, or a food shop, in order to make a choice? There is simply not enough room in my damaged brain to do that any more!

Decision-making is impossible! Finally I buy something but when I get home, I discover that I already have that item in the food cupboard, or this item of clothing does not match anything in my wardrobe. I cannot carry in my brain a register or catalogue of what is at home in order to shop and to choose.

Where am I?

Part of our rising levels of anxiety is losing our way, not knowing where we are. I have somehow lost the map in my head, or at least the way it connects to reality around me. So I need you to guide me around, unless I am in very familiar places in the area around my house. Finding my way is now becoming increasingly difficult. When Paul and I go for walks, I hang onto his hand – he is my global positioning system. I usually have no idea where we are, which direction we are going.

In May 2000, I went by myself to a university residential in Bathurst, as part of my counselling diploma. It was a nightmare – I was unable to find my way from the residence, to the dining room, to the lecture room, only a distance of, say, 50 metres each time, and just had to follow familiar faces (of course never familiar names – I had no idea what their names were). It was the last time I tried to go anywhere unfamiliar without a care-partner to guide me.

Communicating

We know what we want, but we can't say it. In my view we are not cognitively impaired but communication impaired. Speaking, reading, writing, numbers have all become scrambled. The wires in our head that once did this all somehow automatically, have now burnt out.

They are misfiring, becoming crossed over, or absent. As a result, our struggle to communicate increases each day.

What is that word I want?

As we speak, gaps in the flow of words appear. In our head a string of pictures has formed, but the words for those pictures no longer make their way into our consciousness, let alone to our mouth. The words for those pictures seem as if they are on a loose spinning wheel. If interrupted, I have to start again, or I simply forget totally what I was going to say. And the thought does not come back later – it is gone for good. My sentences have become more convoluted as I struggle to find the right word, and if the wheel spins too far, the wrong word comes out.

For me, speaking is always a struggle now, so I am slower and more confused in what I say. It is as if my shelves of neatly filed words have been swept off onto the floor, and I have to search among untidy heaps to find the word I am looking for. If I find it, or its nearest equivalent, I then have to work out how to pronounce it and where to put it in a sentence. I give up. Most of the time I use the word 'Thingy' which describes anything I have forgotten the actual word for! A lady who used to be a teacher said 'My adjectives are disappearing – and I used to be so strong in using them.'

My sentences come out very scrambled, and I come out with odd things – like saying, 'You'll need some more cereal water' instead of 'milk'. I am describing the word because the wheel has not spun to give me the correct term, only the description. Or the wires are crossed over in my brain and the wrong word comes out altogether, like the time I said to my daughter, 'Let's go and plant the horses', and we both doubled up with laughter realising what had happened. I had seen the horse when thinking about planting trees. Then there was the time when I yelled out to Paul, 'Oh my goodness, the long thing is rushing around everywhere!' meaning 'the hose is on the ground gushing water'.

A real difficulty in speaking is words like 'we', 'they', 'I', 'you', 'he' – when I have to work out who is doing what to whom. It simply is so hard, and doesn't seem to make sense in my head. I talk about our family finances as 'my' money, 'my' bills, 'my' tax, even though we have joint accounts and everything is shared between us.

But when I meet someone outside the family, I speak very slowly, and use all my focus and effort to appear normal. I am like a high-wire act in a circus, needing lots of concentration otherwise I'll fall off. A long chat with you, and I'm exhausted and sore in the head afterwards. With the family I have a safety net for my high-wire act, and I can relax and just try to communicate my thoughts and feelings as best I can. It all comes out very muddled, but the family do their best to mind-read!

As we write, the letters come out peculiarly shaped or missing, and what appears on the page can look like an unfamiliar jumble, no longer recognisable as our handwriting. It's like speaking, somehow the right word or tense is suddenly missing in my brain when I need it. But I can bash away at the computer – and get a good laugh from the spell check!

This book took six years to write, and is the result of talks I wrote and gave in this time, emails I wrote and received, and interviews with the media. I cut and pasted all of this material and then tried very hard to put it all together to make sense. Through doing this, I had time to share my thoughts slowly, reiteratively and reflectively.

Reading is becoming increasingly difficult, following the lines on the page, and remembering the names and the story. But I have easy-to-read books, and work at it, so I am still able to read. I just must never stop, it seems, nor even slow down! I try to use a card under the lines to keep my eyes tracking the page. And of course when I turn the page, I have forgotten the last few lines, so flip the page back and forth to get the flow of words into my head. I try to note down things, and keep re-reading sections. There is a big problem of thought-sequencing, where I can't hold onto the ideas, names or concepts long enough to understand them.

Mostly I skim read, as otherwise I can't grasp the thread of the story. If I go too slow, I forget what has just gone before, so I need to go fast to make the story somehow hang together. It seems as if there are just too many words to put together and make sense, and not enough space inside my head to sort the words into a story and to hang onto it long enough to follow the plot.

It's like I have a patchwork mind, reading in patches, then trying to put it all together. My brain is like a sieve, with facts falling through the holes. I need to read fast, as if I'm impatient and in a hurry, to stop them all falling through the cracks. It is an exhausting way to read, and I can really understand how friends of mine with dementia say they have forgotten their glasses, or are no longer interested in reading. It is one more huge effort in our daily struggle. Writing is the same – intense concentration on each thought, quickly getting it onto paper or computer, and then later skim reading to try to make it into a coherent whole.

I shared some of my feelings and struggles with reading with my friends in DASNI, saying, 'I could read an article, putting bits and pieces together, and more or less making sense of it. But to follow the lines and thread of a long story line in a book – especially turning a page – was really worrying and not possible. I lost patience, was too agitated, and lost the plot.'

I then outlined some of my strategies and struggles with very simple books, and how I had given up on Solzhenitsyn's *Gulag Archipelago*. John from the US wrote 'I got so tired of making notes of story lines, which character was which. I'd have to do this each night after reading a little. I just gave up…your posting was so valid in my case about saying, "I'm too busy to read", when it's really the frustration of trying to follow the story, rereading the same page a couple of times.'[28] And Jan said, 'You are able to put [this] into words so easily…I will try your approach. Thanks for the tip.'[29]

The wisdom of Morris then inspired me to keep up the struggle, when he wrote 'I hope you get back to *Gulag*, Christine. Solzhenitsyn can inspire us to survive (one day at a time) the dementia Gulag (Soviet prison camp)… My secret is skimming and feeling free to skim.'[30]

Numbers get all muddled up!

Calculating has become another hurdle. We struggle to write numbers, line them up and do simple arithmetic. We simply cannot remember what we are supposed to do. What does an eight mean, really? What does it mean to say two times two? Where inside your head does twenty take away seven happen?

Telephone numbers get disordered as I write them down, so I cannot be relied upon to transcribe a number. I misdial long numbers for overseas or mobiles. It takes a longer time to dial the number and the phone often cuts out. Multiplying or trying to manipulate numbers makes little sense, and I'm back to adding up and subtracting, and even then it's a struggle. But I keep practising, keep trying to check our bank statements, and using a calculator, to keep some level of skill.

Isolation

Isolation is a real problem for us. Many of us feel that some people even think dementia is contagious! We don't see many friends any more. It seems as if people treat us differently now, because they know we have dementia, and they don't know what to do. Maybe they are worried about us saying something odd or doing something bizarre? Often we feel like we are being watched in case we do the wrong thing.

People with dementia often talk about friends and extended family continuing to visit for a while after diagnosis, but then no longer coming. One fellow said: 'They get upset when we lose our train of thought, or leap in with the answer to the question because we can't get the answer out quickly enough.'

But it is an issue for our care-partners too. I have heard one lady say, 'I am so busy being busy, remembering for two, doing everything around the house. When do I get time to socialise? Friends offer to help but they really don't understand what it is like.'

There are many ways to help

I think the important thing to remember about dementia is that the symptoms we show are the result of several things working together, some of which you can address. Firstly there is the brain pathology, the damage that is occurring day by day. At the moment there is little that can be done, except in cases of vascular dementia where low-dose aspirin may reduce the likelihood of further damage. Let's all work together to encourage research for a cure so that one day we can stop the damage.

Other important factors influencing the way we react to this brain damage, and so exhibit the symptoms of dementia, are our personality and our life story. This is the same in many illnesses, as our attitude truly determines how we tackle major issues in our lives. So it is with dementia: how we cope with this struggle into increasing problems with thinking, memory and physical functioning often depends on how we have coped with problems in our past life. You can help here by building on our strengths, working with reminiscence, and most importantly by trying to understand what this assault to our functioning is like.

Then there is our environment, and there is plenty you can do to manage this, whether we are at home or in residential care. I talk about this later in this section.

We should try to rekindle and remember (there's an irony) our memories through photo albums and life histories. Let's keep up with friends, books, films, church, whatever gave us these memories. But let's also create new ones. Days out, travel, gardening, sport, reading, shared time – as long as we want to do these things, whatever we want to do. And let's remember those things too, our more immediate history and life story. Keep that camera handy.

That's not easy for people who have spent many years together, who are probably overwhelmed by loss. But life is not all in the past. *Carpe diem*, let's seize the day – together. It doesn't really matter if I don't remember today or don't know what day of the week it is. As long as we all enjoyed it to the fullest together.

Finally, and in many ways most importantly, there is our underlying spirituality. This is not simply what religion we might practise; it is what has given us meaning in our lives. Maybe it is our garden, our art or our pets. It may well be familiar rituals of our religion. It is important for you to help us reconnect with what has given us meaning as we journey deeper into the centre of our being, into our spirit.

We can live in the present, treasuring each moment, and it is important for us to feel peace around us. A beautiful garden or the delights of nature can capture this peace, much as a bud expresses the full potential of life.

Get the right diagnosis

The first step to helping us is to make sure we get the right diagnosis, and that we are followed up regularly. There are around 70 causes of dementia. Of course, many are quite rare, but all too often a diagnosis of Alzheimer's is given, with the assumption made that the person will deteriorate rapidly according to expectations. And often that is the case, because depression sets in. This is hardly surprising, given the nature of the diagnosis. Depression is an excellent mimic of dementia – and for many the diagnosis is truly the beginning of the end, and a self-fulfilling prophecy – possibly much of the deterioration in the early stages is due to depression.

But we should be much more cautious, and more willing to recognise that the brain is a very individual organ, and each person responds to brain damage in a different way. Not all dementias are Alzheimer's, nor are all cases of Alzheimer's similar in the way they affect the person. This is important, as treatment and management vary according to the disease. We need to be careful in making a diagnosis, and to encourage people and remind them that they are an individual, with a unique way of handling any disease, particularly this one.

Fronto-temporal dementia is under-diagnosed, as is Lewy Body dementia – often in older people Alzheimer's is the catch-all label used. In younger people the opposite occurs. I know someone who was initially told she was menopausal, but she has Lewy Body dementia. Another friend was told he had Parkinson's, but his difficulties in working out how to put a tape into the car stereo were because of cognition not muscular control.

In support groups I have been to, one issue frequently talked about was the lack of interest and support from local doctors. I gave a talk in 2001, in the offices of a local medical association. This had been organised by the Alzheimer's Association. There was excellent preparation, promotion, snacks, professional video, a speaker – but no audience. Not a single doctor came to that evening's talk, so I spoke to the video camera. It was a poignant and powerful reminder of just what is wrong with the local doctors.

Our doctors need to be alert to the early signs of dementia, and to be up to date with treatment strategies. It is important that people are carefully assessed, and referred by their doctor to a specialist who is prepared to follow up every three to six months until a more certain diagnosis can be made. And then they should be seen every six months to a year.

If I had simply accepted my initial diagnosis of Alzheimer's Disease, I could have certainly subsided into major depression and been put into a nursing home as a consequence – where I would have remained depressed. And what if I had not been prescribed medication? Now that I have been followed up since my initial diagnosis, it is quite astounding how unexpected the outcome has been. I believe much of this is due to the attitude of my neurologist who observes me as an individual with unique responses to brain damage. Also I had a careful and methodical local doctor who referred me very quickly to this neurologist. Now I am blessed to have a really good local doctor who reviews my functioning and medication regularly, and refers me for annual check-ups.

Treatment delayed is treatment denied

As soon as a diagnosis of dementia is given, treatment and support should start. Why are many of us not offered treatment? Often we are just told the 'dementia script' of decline then death, and given no hope. There is hope after a diagnosis of dementia. It is possible to live positively.

Anti-dementia drugs, such as the cholinesterase inhibitors, should be offered as soon as possible after diagnosis. They can help what remains to work better, but they do not stop the damage. It is vital to take medication as early as possible, because function we lose is not easily regained. Treatment delayed is effectively treatment denied, as we will have lost function forever. The drugs can stabilise our symptoms for periods of at least six months to a year, and in some cases a lot longer, giving us valuable time at home to enjoy each day while we can still do a great deal. They won't make us live longer, but may delay our entry into a nursing home.

There was an alarming time for me in August 2000, when I switched straight across to 10 mg of Donepazil (Aricept), from the maximum dose of Tacrine. These were both anti-dementia drugs, but worked in a different way. I had a difficult month of adjustment, and I wrote about my struggle to my friends in DASNI:

> Thanks everyone for your support. I'm having 'down time' at the moment. My brain feels like a huge ball of cotton wool got in there, my eyes feel swollen and tired, and my legs feel like lead. I'm trying to adjust to Aricept (10 mg) having switched over on Sat after five years on 160 mg of Cognex (Tacrine). I just hope I bounce back soon.[31]

It took a while, but I did bounce back, from the fuzziness of confusion, and eventually was able to recover a level of functioning that allowed me to enjoy each day. Aricept, and before that, Cognex, has made an enormous difference to my quality of life, keeping me able to function to my full potential. I now also take Ebixa (Memantine). Without my tablets, it is like thinking in fog and walking in treacle.

Without these medicines, I would not be able to speak or write, let alone produce this book! I would be very slow, tired and confused. With my 'battery charger' – as I call it – I can enjoy a full day as long as I am never under any stress. It raises the levels of a type of chemical messenger, acetyl choline, in my brain, so there are more chances of signals getting through in my brain. It does not stop the brain damage, nor cure the disease, but without it I seem to wind down, no longer able to speak, think or do much at all.

For many people these drugs help in daily functioning, making the mind clearer and activities easier – even sleeping can be much improved. One lady I know noticed these changes days after starting Aricept, and we certainly notice her improved ability to use her diary and calendar to keep her life organised. She was there, at home, when we arrived to give her a lift to the support group, instead of out walking her dog, having forgotten completely about the group.

Other medication should also be offered, particularly for depression and vascular disease where appropriate. And we need to know about alternative medicines such as Vitamins E and C, lecithin and gingko biloba that have been shown to help address brain damage.

Try to understand how hard it is for us

Remember that our odd behaviour and memory difficulties are the result of a physical disease. Husbands and wives of people with dementia have said, 'She or he doesn't seem to want to do something, doesn't seem to try very hard, is being awkward or difficult, just watches TV, doesn't really do gardening, just potters, not like before.' All sorts of negative comments. We try to remind them that their loved one is trying very hard, it's just that you can't see the missing bits that they are having to cope without.

We say, 'If they had a missing arm or leg, you'd be very proud of the way they are managing, and they are trying just so hard to cope, and should be praised for their efforts. It's not easy to realise how much effort they are making in simply living each day, and how this physical damage is causing the problems you are seeing.'

When I asked people with dementia whether families realised how hard they were trying to cope, they said, 'No, because you look normal but you're not, and it's a real struggle just to get through each day.' And when I asked whether their family really understands, the response was 'No, not really. They think I am not trying hard enough. And sometimes they expect too much of me, but at other times I am not allowed to do what I am capable of. I am not allowed to choose what I can or cannot do. But then sometimes it is easier to walk away, than to argue that I can do something.'

Above all, please remember we are individual human beings. We have dementia, and you can't see the damage, so you don't know what it is like. Don't assume too much. Take us at face value, as a person, first and foremost, not a disease. Then help us to keep on achieving to our full potential.

Value us, give us dignity

How you relate to us has a big impact on the course of the disease. You can restore our personhood, and give us a sense of being needed and valued. There is a Zulu saying that is very true, 'A person is a person through others.'[32] Give us reassurance, hugs, support, a meaning in life. Value us for what we can still do and be, and make sure we retain social networks. It is very hard for us to be who we once were, so let us be who we are now – and realise the effort we are making to function. If you could see the damage inside our head, you would be amazed at the way we are managing despite missing bits in our brain.

Include us in the activities of community organisations, particularly those addressing dementia. Are we on your committees, boards, seminar organising groups and suchlike? Unlike people with other diseases, we seem to be written off from active participation in addressing our own needs.

I was greatly encouraged to get an email from Professor Steven Sabat of Georgetown University, Washington, D.C. He is writing about how people with dementia can become active participants in the research process, not merely research subjects.[33] He says in his paper, 'One way to help the person with AD construct a worthy, valued, social persona is to engage said person as a collaborator in research efforts of which there are many types... It is through such research efforts that we may find some pathways not only toward providing people with AD another means by which to construct worthy, valued, social identities, but also toward the unearthing of new knowledge and perspectives about the nature of AD and its cognitive and social effects.'

It is also important to think about our lack of ability to speak. In what way does this limit you in valuing us, in giving us dignity and personal space. I know that when I am no longer able to speak, I could become violent quite easily. People make you do things that you don't want to do, and you have no word for 'No, thank you.' So all you can do is push them out of the way because they want to shower or dress you, or give you food you don't like.

We need to be given the same choices as you, even though we cannot tell you clearly what choice we want to make. And we should not be forced into a pattern of behaviour that simply suits the nursing home, or your own ideas of what we should be doing. Think of us as an individual, not just a care-recipient.

Several times, after my talks, I have been asked 'What should I do if the person doesn't want to get out of their pyjamas in the morning?' I usually say, 'What do you do on a Sunday morning? Do you always get dressed? Do you still sometimes want to go back to bed? Or walk around the house in your pyjamas? Does it really matter that he's still in his pyjamas?'

The world goes much faster than we do, whizzing around, and we are being asked to do things, or to respond, or to play a game, or to participate in group activities. It is too fast, we want to say 'Go away, slow down, leave me alone, just go away', and maybe we might then be difficult, not cooperative.

This is called 'challenging behaviour'. Well, I believe that this is 'adaptive behaviour', where I am adapting to my care environment. I am pushing you when you want me to have a shower, or spitting out my food because I don't like it, or going to the toilet in the wrong place because I have forgotten where the toilet is, or walking into the wrong person's room because I don't know where my room is. Shower us or bath us at a familiar time for us. Find out what food we like. Leave the toilet in clear view. If we can't read numbers anymore, why not mark our rooms with a distinctive sign or picture, something special to us, like a picture of my cat or my favourite flower.

If the care environment is focused on the person and their needs, none of that so-called 'challenging' behaviour needs to happen.

Find help and support

The human brain has developed over a lifetime of experience, in a variety of environments, and so exhibits its own unique coping mechanisms in the face of internal devastation. The initial struggle with cognitive decline and confusion, followed by the diagnosis of dementia, is a traumatic personal experience. Yet this occurs in a social milieu – in our family, in our community, in the context of all our social relationships. It is also an experience set against our past attitudes and behaviour, and our life story.

We are each so unique, and the brain damage will affect us differently according to our environment and to our history. As we lose our cognitive abilities, our stress threshold is lowered and we react more in accord with our deep-set emotions and our past expectations. We need a great deal of help and support, as we struggle with this decline and an increasing inability to deal with it.

Information and help

At the beginning, information is important and empowering. Tell us about the diagnosis, about how little is known, and how individual each one of us is. Refer us to the local Alzheimer's association for information and support about dementia. Provide help sheets for us. We need to understand the nature of this disease, how it is as individual as we are, and that there are many things we can do to help ourselves.

We often need help around the home, particularly if we live alone – and we do want to remain independent for as long as possible. First, we need access to transport – not complicated public transport systems in which we will get confused and lost, but lifts in cars, taxis, buses.

Help us plan for the future

A main issue for people with dementia in my experience is being a
burden to their family, and they want to talk about future care issues,
such as legal and funeral arrangements. Unfortunately they often feel
that they couldn't talk about these issues because it might upset family
members.

When Michelle, the Executive Director of the Alzheimer's Association in Canberra, ran a workshop for families, ten families partici-
pated. Seven families went home and discussed future care arrangements, looked at residential facilities, made wills and even discussed
what sort of funeral they would like.

Later, a husband caring for his wife who was about to be admitted
to residential care thanked Michelle for giving both him and his wife
'permission' to discuss these very important and sensitive topics while
she still could. He feels comfortable with his decision knowing that he
and his wife planned for this day together.

Offer us legal help as soon as possible after our diagnosis, because
we have a terminal illness and need to get our affairs in order. I
arranged an enduring power of attorney, giving me peace of mind.
This document, or a living will or advanced directive, allows us to
exercise our own choices about our future. It may well reassure us
about our financial affairs.

However, it will of course distress us to realise that one day we may
lose our ability to read, write and use numbers. For some of us this
occurs very early on in the disease, yet for others it may be a lot later.

Importantly, we need to be regarded as legally competent until or
unless at least two doctors have carefully assessed us and recommended otherwise. We are 'innocent until proven guilty'. We have full
capacity until it has been proven otherwise. We are each individuals,
with different patterns of disease, and must be assessed accordingly.

Emotional support

In our crisis of identity and our fragmentation, we need you to
acknowledge who we are, to listen to our emotion and pain, and to

treat us a people of value and dignity, worthy of respect. The fear of future decline is a terrible thing to live with. It's a curse that leads to its own fulfilment. The future looks bleak to the person with dementia – it not only looks bleak, but actually is bleak. So I believe it is wrong to deny us help to deal with the whole gamut of emotions we will experience along the journey of their disease.

We need all the support we can get, after having what I think is one of the worst diagnoses anyone can get. Before diagnosis the person worries they are going crazy. There may well be much greater tension in their family relationships as their behaviour deteriorates – and yet expectations of them do not change. The person feels stressed, tired and puzzled as to what is wrong with them. The diagnosis itself may produce feelings of great relief – they are not going mad after all. And their families suddenly realise there is an explanation for the difficulties they have been having. But it is still a crisis. This is a terrible and terrifying diagnosis, a shameful one.

The person then begins to experience anger, suspiciousness, frustration, anxiety, sadness, hopelessness, helplessness and self-blame. And some people experience denial as a way of coping with the crisis of diagnosis – it can't be true!

Grief is one of the first and most common reactions to dementia, and it is an anticipatory loss of self that is being grieved for. The responses to this grief may be mistaken as being a sign of the dementia, yet the following are normal reactions to loss: sadness, anger, anxiety, fatigue, helplessness and shock, disbelief, confusion and preoccupation with thoughts about the disease, sleep disturbance, appetite changes, absent mindedness, social withdrawal and crying.

One thing that can't be overemphasised is the complex, overwhelming, often obscure and gradual, yet irregular progression of losses that occur in dementia. We need to grieve many times, as each successive loss becomes apparent to us. It is so hard to be continually experiencing loss and grief.

In many cases depression sets in, including a loss of self-esteem, where everything feels poor and empty. There is a feeling of horror of what might lie ahead. This is particularly true when the person is treated in accord with the medical model for dementia, with a prognosis of inexorable cognitive decline until death.

Depression may result in 'excess disability', giving rise to cognitive and memory problems additional to those of the disease process. It is an excellent mimic of dementia, and needs to be treated, so that the person does not experience an excess disability, and become even more fearful and confused, entering a vicious spiral downward into worsening symptoms of dementia and depression.

Denial is a normal reaction to grief, and yet for the person with dementia it is often regarded as a 'lack of insight'. Those in denial are often less anxious and less depressed, so maybe it is an adaptive response to the grief caused by deteriorating function. For example, if I think nothing is wrong with me, and ignore what I feel, then there is nothing to process, nothing to get anxious about, nothing to get depressed about.

Anxiety and fear become more prevalent as the disease progresses, and psychotic symptoms begin to be shown. In the early stages, maybe we can use our earlier learnt coping skills to manage the anxiety generated by our deteriorating function and disorientation, but eventually our internal resources are unable to cope, and the anxiety is expressed as a 'catastrophic reaction'. This physical behaviour is often referred to as 'challenging', but is usually the only means left for us to express our anxiety and emotion, and the distress we are experiencing due to our care environment.

Delusions and hallucinations may occur during the course of dementia. But again, let's not be too ready to use a medical approach, treating these psychotic reactions like those occurring in mental illness. They may indeed be another adaptive response, as the person with dementia struggles to interpret a world which is now experienced as increasingly chaotic as dementia progresses. Can their environment be made more simple more secure, more comforting, less distressing?

Paranoia and psychosis may well be perfectly logical responses to what is happening around us, given our memory difficulties, our intermittent reception of what you say, and our fear of not being in control.

We misinterpret our environment, and try to make sense of it to restore our feelings of order.

The key question is what can be done for the person with a diagnosis of dementia who starts along this path of disturbed emotions and behaviour. Drugs are of course useful for depression, but the debate continues as to the usefulness of anti-psychotic drugs for what are euphemistically called 'challenging behaviours'. At best they may be modestly effective.

Provide specialised counselling for us, as well as support groups if we would like to go to these. Or maybe we can use 'cyberspace', like in DASNI, where we can socialise at times when we feel like it and not be public or confronted, simply sharing privately with others via our computer how we feel. These groups can give us an environment in which we feel normal, in which we no longer need to hide the fact that we have dementia. We need to know we are not the only one that feels this way. If there isn't a group, help set one up!

We need emotional support, especially immediately after diagnosis. Listen to our anger and grief, and help us to deal with emotional issues from the past and with our grief at what we will lose in the future.

Empowerment and hope

Don't assume we are depressed simply because we aren't as active as we once were. People with dementia often say they are not depressed, yet their family thinks they are. Is this because the care-partners are themselves feeling depressed, so if they are depressed then surely their husband, wife, mother, father must be depressed as well? Or is it a lack of understanding that the person with dementia needs time out to rest and cannot maintain the same level of participation as before. One family member commented, 'He just sits and gazes into space.' Is this depression or someone who just needs time to recharge their batteries? Maybe it is very hard to understand how the vibrant, energetic person you once knew is now someone who doesn't participate as actively as they once did in everything happening around them.

In many ways, the experience of dementia and its diagnosis is like a chronic trauma, and our feelings are similar – of disempowerment and disconnection from others. Often the result of chronic trauma is post-traumatic stress disorder, characterised by withdrawal, numbness, apathy, irritability, emotional outbursts and impaired memory and concentration.

If people with dementia have excess disability resulting from post-traumatic stress disorder, maybe they could be helped to overcome some of these reactions. I developed this thinking in an article I wrote in 2001[34] and suggested that treatment strategies should aim to empower us, encourage the creation of relationships, and restore the capacity for trust, autonomy, initiative, competence, identity and intimacy.

Morris, in an email to DASNI in early 2001, agreed, saying, 'Post-traumatic stress disorder results from a dreadful experience or catastrophe outside the range of normal human experience. The combination of having a progressive incurable terminal dementing disease and being diagnosed with it certainly qualifies.'[35]

I think the key to helping us cope with the trauma of living with dementia is to give us hope. Let us know we are unique, with our own inner resources. We have our life story, which tells how we coped in the past. And this affects how we can cope today. We can try to discover an identity as a survivor of dementia and its diagnosis. Most importantly, encourage us to be positive, to hope for a new life in the slow lane, as we reach for the stars together.

Use it or lose it

We need to focus on enhancing our remaining abilities and compensating for any losses, and maybe even working towards a new perspective of daring to try to recover skills, develop new talents, and create a new future invested with meaning and hope.

Morris has been pioneering in his suggestions of rehabilitation for a person with dementia.[36] He suggests we first need to have hope in order to overcome the trauma, and then to confront the why of the disease. Then we need to think about what abilities we still have, and move on from there in an attitude of child-like play to engage problems, taking only one step at a time in the learning process, and to persevere with the task. He says it is important that we validate ourselves, consolidate achievements through repetition, and look to respite as a reward.

The catch phrase 'use it or lose it' is painfully true in the case of dementia. If we stop doing things, we will rapidly forget these tasks. But the brain is a resourceful organ. Never underestimate its capacity to try to find other ways of doing things.

Make sure we don't give up, but don't overtax us. We will get easily exhausted, and need simple tasks that make us feel good about ourselves. Give us time and space to try to keep doing as much as we can. Don't take over unless you really have to. Let us make mistakes or fail, but don't let us feel a failure. Encourage us and make us feel worthwhile, still useful and valued.

Is there perhaps some way you can help us carry on doing at least some ordinary chores? Maybe signs around the place, colour coding light and other switches, lists each day of steps to take for each task. Don't do it all for us – surely there is something useful we can still do?

We need help keeping our lives organised, being reminded of daily activities, assisted with shopping, cooking, cleaning, dressing, showering etc. But we will not be able to ask for all of this. We do not realise we need it. Present information simply and clearly, with not too many choices, and encourage us to function as a normal human being. Help us make choices in small areas of our lives so that we feel in control, and not pushed into things.

Maybe get us a diary, or simply a short list of things to do each day. A friend in my support group had a poster pinned to his wardrobe door, so that it was the first thing he saw on waking. It said, 'Get up, wash, shave, use deodorant, get dressed.' It reminded him where he was and what to do. Help us parcel out activities for each day, and remind us about the day's activities to get a sense of the day and date, and to register what we did yesterday or last week. Even of we can no longer read, you can talk us through our daily activities.

Perhaps think up some sort of 'brain gym' – reading children's books, magazines, particularly in the early stages, to keep us able to cling on to these abilities. We might want to watch quiz shows, look at newspapers, play board games or do crosswords. We might want to do craft, needlework or art. Perhaps we would rather have walks in crisp autumn leaves, or smell and touch beautiful flowers, or even have the relaxation of massage and aromatherapy.

Maybe the golf club can arrange a buddy to play a round of golf with us and keep our score and find our ball! I know of several keen golfers who developed dementia and were no longer welcomed by their golfing friends as they could no longer keep their score correctly. But they delighted in being accompanied by a volunteer through the Alzheimer's Association who assisted them.

Another idea might be to help us to develop our life story, with photos, business cards, favourite foods and so on, so that we enjoy recapturing memories and have a resource alongside us as the disease progresses.

But the key to all of this must be to make the most of our limited energy budget. Please don't try to make us do too much, or what is really beyond our ability. What is the point of testing us to see if we know the date, for example, as this will make us uncomfortably aware of what we cannot do? What we need are a few selected activities that help us feel that we can still accomplish things that are enjoyable and meaningful for us.

Why wear us out with lots of activities, when maybe there is just one thing that we would really like to do each day. One thing that would make a difference in our life, and perhaps also in the lives of others. Find out what our real priority is, and then manage our life by helping with all sorts of other things so that we can focus on that one thing we want to do.

Paul does a lot of the household tasks, such as cooking, washing, shopping, planning and helping to write a list of things to do each day. He also represents us at dementia groups, church activities, and other things we are involved with. Now Paul is taking over the burden of planning, organising and responding to requests, following up correspondence, and reducing my activities in the dementia area. I have asked him to do this to avoid my catastrophic stress reactions, when I cannot sleep, when I shout or cry, when I feel unable to cope even with the most simple enquiry.

I try to spend time with my daughters, listening to them and sharing the important moments in their lives, as well as to try to keep in touch with my DASNI friends, and make this last effort to share about my journey with dementia. Paul has freed me to focus my limited energy on what really matters to me.

Morris made this point very clearly, when he shared with DASNI, 'One pet point I'd like to see made is 'choose your battles'...[we] function as well as we do because we are very conscious of and respectful of fatigue. So often advice is blandly given to exercise the brain, and the person wastes their precious resources on crossword puzzles or trivial conversation rather than thinking thoughts that count.'[37]

We can learn new things, in this journey to focus on what is important, and what gives us a sense of meaning and self-worth. I have spoken to my friends with dementia about this, whether they could think of any positives from our diagnosis with dementia. Some talked of time to be with family or animals, others about new challenges they were able to take up, and about the healing of relationships.

In Christchurch, we all sat round as a group, and Frank Drysdale from Australia amazed us all by sharing how he had an inspiration from God to develop the game Numero, complete with the ideas and rules for the game.[38] It has been a great success in education worldwide, and the profits have been donated to the Western Australia Alzheimer's Association. God can give us gifts and we need to use them despite our dementia, and we may be able to help others even in a small way.

I have learnt how to use PowerPoint for my talks, so have a major sense of achievement. It took me a long time, and I am limited in my use, but I feel good about myself. It has also been an excellent tool for communicating about living with dementia, visually and with words, in other languages and cultures. It is something I can point to as a positive outcome of living with dementia.

All this effort at the computer, to try to keep reading, to keep active in my thinking – it's a bit like I'm a 'brain athlete' from doing all those exercises. I'm keeping my brain working with a great deal of effort. Maybe it's a bit like being a wheelchair athlete, in that I feel as if I have a very muscled 115-year-old brain. The anti-dementia drug bathes my brain in a chemical messenger so that all the signals are much more active, so could be called a 'brain steroid'!

But of course, I can't keep up this effort all the time. There are some days when I say 'It is all too hard. Why can't I just forget everything, forget taking the tablets, just be at home and rest!' I find each day is such a struggle. I'm sure athletes feel like that too, like giving up. Then I think about the people with dementia that I see in day-care centers and nursing homes, and the struggles they are having because they can't tell people what their world is like, so I have kept going, just one more day at a time, to try to share what it is like for us.

Communicating with us

Touching our emotion and spirit

As we become more emotional and less cognitive, it's the way you talk to us, not what you say, that we will remember. We know the feeling, but don't know the plot. Your smile, your laugh and your touch are what we will connect with. Empathy heals. Just love us as we are. Visit us and just be with us if you do not know what to say. We don't need words so much as your presence, your sharing of feelings with us. We're still here, in emotion and spirit, if only you could find us!

We need you to listen carefully as we can't repeat our words. We struggle to speak and it often comes out in a very scrambled way, without proper grammar and syntax. Please try to make sense of the feelings we are trying to convey. The sense of being listened to, and of being heard, will make us feel valued and in a relationship with you. This is what we need as we cope with shattered thoughts and fragmented selves.

One thing at a time

I operate in a different way to you, and need a different type of interaction, which is slower and more meaningful. People want to be busy, to talk fast, to ask for responses, but I can't cope with that. I need a restful, calm environment, with no visual or aural distraction, to listen to what you say and to be able to speak to you.

I won't be able to concentrate on what you are saying and will get very confused, so I need quiet time to restore my energy. Please don't play music or have the TV on when you are talking to me. If the TV is on, please mute it first before talking to us. We won't realise we need you to do this, though, and may even complain. But one source of sound is usually enough!

Connecting with us

Just because we can't express ourselves very well does not mean we have nothing to say. As our thoughts and words are tangled and confused, you will need good listening skills, being attentive to non-verbal cues. Take what we say in context, as the words and their order will be wrong. Try to find the meaning behind the words as we will make mistakes in tenses, words and grammar. Be sure we would like you to help fill in the gaps in our struggle to find words and sentences before you do so. Don't correct us, just try to understand the meaning of what we intend to say.

Don't interrupt our thread of thought, but let us interrupt you when an idea comes into our head, because if we wait, it will disappear. Try the technique of reflective listening, where you repeat back what we have said to you, not exactly, but repeat the meaning of what we have tried to say. This will help ensure you have understood our true meaning, and help us feel really listened to.

Give us time to speak, wait for us to find the word we want to use, and don't let us feel embarrassed if we lose the thread of what we say. I remember one friend, George (not his real name) walking tentatively into the room where we had recently started a small coffee group for people with dementia, as an alternative to the day care centre. His wife was most anxious about how he would cope with a 'talking group' as apparently he could not really communicate any more, and might feel upset in this group.

We started chatting about this and that, over a cup of coffee and some biscuits. Soon I noticed George had sat a bit forward, and his lip quivered, and he looked as if he wanted to say something. So I asked the others to stop for a moment, and said 'I think George wants to tell us something. Go ahead, it's OK, you've got plenty of time. We know what it's like to try to find words.' And we just sat in silence for a while, as he gathered his thoughts, and slowly started to speak. Every now and then, we would stop talking again to give him the space in which to speak and to be heard.

His wife came to collect him, and walked to the car, helped him in, and then came rushing back inside. She gave me a big hug, and was delighted. George had told her that he had enjoyed the morning and since then he has gone again to the group a few times, and then on to the day care centre which he had avoided before. Maybe we had helped him feel less alone, more accepted, and given him permission to feel words were difficult and confusing.

Try to avoid direct questions, which can alarm us or make us feel very uncomfortable. Questions also make us feel pressured for the immediacy we have lost. If we have forgotten something special that happened recently, don't assume we didn't enjoy it. Just give us a gentle prompt – we may just be momentarily blank. Even if we never remember, surely the memory of the event is not what is important – it is our experience at the time that really matters.

It is best to look at us, to make sure there is eye contact and that we are attending from the beginning of what you say. Speak clearly and not too fast. Slow down when you speak, so we can follow you, for we will have gaps in reception and understanding – and the faster that you talk, the more we will miss. Don't shout at us, though – the problem is often not our hearing, but our understanding. Shouting simply distresses us – for me it feels as if you are hitting my head, causing even more confusion inside there.

Most importantly, don't push us into something, because we can't think or speak fast enough to let you know whether we agree. Try to give us time to respond – to let you know whether we really want to do it. Being forced into things makes us upset or aggressive, even fearful.

Look behind our behaviour to its meaning, as we communicate with you in this way. You can enter our reality, accept more emotion and feeling, and connect with us at this level as our cognition fails and inhibitions decrease.

Touching us, to connect with us, may be helpful. Many of us may not like to be touched by people we do not know, but find it therapeutic to be touched by people we do know. Stroking is an important part of touch, and I find it lovely to touch and to stroke, and to be touched, to connect in this way.

When in Japan, I visited a day care centre in Matsue, and it was lovely to kneel in front of each person, take them by the hand, look them in the eye, and speak quietly with them. Even the lady who could not speak or see squeezed my hand in recognition of my presence. She was communicating with me in that way.

Observing us will be the key to knowing what we are saying to you. Most of our communication is non-verbal. Our facial expressions, our hand gestures, and the context in which we are trying to communicate with you are all important. How will you know that we are in pain when we can no longer speak? What if I have earache and can't tell you? With my cat, I can tell when her ear hurts by looking at her behaviour – she might shake her head, have her head on one side, and look miserable. She has 'told' me all I need to know about her earache.

Goldsmith has summarised beautifully how to improve communication with people with dementia:

- provide a restful environment
- be calm, reassuring and relaxed
- approach the person within their line of vision and identify yourself, maintaining eye contact at the same level
- use touch where acceptable to the person

- speak simply and slowly, but respectfully
- allow time for understanding
- be a good listener, allow pauses and look for meaning behind words
- use short sentences without double messages
- illustrate what you are saying where possible, with aids such as photos
- try to follow what they are saying, do not correct mistakes nor laugh at inappropriate responses
- be complimentary where appropriate
- do not be embarrassed by displays of emotion.[39]

Living with stigma

Do what you can to prevent the stigma of dementia. We people with dementia have two burdens from our disease. The first is the struggle with the illness itself. The second is the battle we have with what I call the 'disease of society'. Dementia, and the type of dementia called Alzheimer's, are a disease of society as much as they are a disease of a person.

Hazel Hawke, former 'first lady' in Australia, who has been diagnosed with Alzheimer's Disease, said, 'Ridicule is terribly hurtful to the sufferer and it doesn't serve any purpose... Alzheimer's...is kind of shameful, it's embarrassing, you're losing your marbles.'[40]

Stigma is a social issue separating the world into two perceived compartments, by labelling and lack of understanding: that of dementia, and that of 'normals'. This is the stigma we face, where the stereotype and myths surrounding dementia perpetuate an attitude that isolates us, into a separate, walled compartment of dementia.

Until this wall created by stigma is removed, people will not seek help, nor even seek a diagnosis, and then they will be denied the treatment and support that is available to them. Living with dementia, we need to be free of stigma to feel respected and empowered, and to know we can live a new life in the slow lane.

I found that when I read a book describing the difficulties of people with mental disability by James Dudley, I could easily replace 'intellectual disability' with the word dementia.[41] We too 'live within a complex web of social encounters that are tainted with stigma... [which] like racism is pervasive and endemic to [our] existence'.

Our world becomes circumscribed by the stigma of our illness. We want to retreat in shame, and do not want to 'come out' and tell people the diagnosis. It's not surprising that some of us react by denying anything is wrong, and our families do too. Better to pretend at normalcy than to face up to the challenge of dementia.

If we do believe the lie of dementia, that we can't learn new things, remember anything reliably, or find our way around, we are blind-folded to our own potential. We withdraw into helplessness and let our families take over. Our inner world is in turmoil as we suffer antici-patory grief at loss of self. We may become overwhelmed by feelings of anxiety, anger, sadness, fatigue, shock, helplessness and numbness as we try to come to terms with losing ourselves as well as others.

Please don't call us 'dementing' – we are still people separate from our disease, we just have a disease of the brain. If I had cancer you would not refer to me as 'cancerous', would you?

Our labels seem to mean so much – am I Alzheimer's Disease or fronto-temporal dementia, or simply someone with a 'dementing illness'? All these terms label us as someone without capacity, without credibility as a member of the community. How about separating us from the illness in some way? How about remembering we are a person with progressive brain damage?

Be very alert for discrimination against people with dementia. Treat us like a normal person and never speak about us in the third person when we are there. Don't criticise, find fault or laugh at us, or speak as if we are no longer there, and certainly do not do everything for us. Respect us and realise how hard we are trying to cope.

Don't categorise us in terms of stages of the disease. This is mean-ingless at the individual level. Our cortex is wired up according to our own unique learning and experience, so we vary in how we react to damage in any area of our brain. We need to be treated as an individual, with unique capabilities.

Focus on our abilities not our deficiencies. Treat us as a person, never a statistic, and involve us in life. Help us to continue activities that we enjoy – whatever will help us to feel valued, appreciated, and still part of society.

Dementia-friendly environment

Our environment is a critical part of our disease. How we exhibit symptoms will very much depend on our environment and how well we can cope with it. We need love, comfort, attachment, inclusion, identity and occupation as our world around us becomes strange and our ability scrambled.

The importance of the person's environment in coping with the experience of dementia has been the focus of work by Kitwood[42] who made a detailed study of the impact on the manifestation of dementia related to the institutional care environment. He suggested that dementia arises from a complex interaction between various factors unique to the person, which would explain the great variability of symptoms and progression of losses that accompany any particular type of dementia in different people.

First there is the personality, or resources for action, including a set of avoidances and blocks acquired through life's experiences of failure, fear or powerlessness, accompanied by various defences against anxiety. Next is the biography, or life story, including all losses and current social support. Then there is physical health, including sensory function, which may affect the degree of confusion and ability to communicate. These all affect the way the person copes with the actual brain damage.

The most important factor for improving care is the environment, as this can be changed quite easily to ensure that it enhances the person's sense of safety, value and well being. It needs to validate the person's experiences and emotions, facilitate the person's actions, celebrate the person's abilities, and provide sensory pleasures.

But sometimes the family home is where past conflicts, present tensions and well-worn patterns of behaviour may profoundly affect the expression of dementia. Please try to make sure you get help, to address any underlying emotional issues. As emotional beings, we are buffeted by our environment, with few cognitive resources to cope with stress. So we are very susceptible to our environment and to any family dysfunction. We cannot cope with stress, tension, arguments or unease around us.

As environment is so important to the expression of dementia, there is a great deal you can do to help. How we exhibit symptoms will very much depend on how well we can cope as the world around us becomes strange and our ability scrambled. Our behaviour is usually a perfectly reasonable response to our environment given the degree of brain damage we have.

Avoid background noise, which will make me tired and confused, anxious and even aggressive. A quiet environment helps avoid additional confusion. I wonder why so many day care centres and nursing homes have a TV, radio and talking all happening at once? No wonder the people sitting there look so blank! Maybe think about ear plugs for a visit to shopping centres or other noisy places.

If children are underfoot, remember we will get tired very easily and find it very hard to concentrate on talking or listening as well. Make sure we face away from any visual disturbances, and that we are in a quiet place.

Encourage routine so that we can feel safe and secure in a familiar environment, with a set of activities that we can recall. This will reduce the stress of trying to make sense of our surroundings.

Make our spaces uncluttered, particularly in areas like the kitchen and bathroom. Use a combined shampoo and conditioner so there are not too many bottles. Try to have a shower that is easy to get into, and a tap that only has one control, and no very hot or cold water.

We may have difficulty in vision and coordination which mean we might knock things over and feel clumsy. Decanting things into plastic containers might avoid breakages. If we do knock things over, and stare blankly at the mess we have made, please help us clear up, as we can't think through the steps needed, and get flustered and confused.

The entry and exit doors to toilets in public places, such as community centres, are a real challenge. They never seem to be painted a contrasting colour, so that we can find our way in and out of the toilet. There can be so many doors in there to confuse us, and our care-partner may not be able to go in there to help us. Whenever we have gone out with groups of people with dementia, this is always an issue. Someone is late coming out, and you hear doors banging as someone tries to work out which door is the right way out of the toilet. If only the entry and exit doors were a contrasting colour to all the other doors, we wouldn't get as confused and might be able to go out more often!

Enter our reality

Our reality can become caught between dreams and daily life, because between sleep and awake is another world – a terror-land of illusion, inhabited by dark shapes, real feelings, but an inability to move, or speak, or escape. So what is real, what is true?

Dreams are very vivid, because our sleeping mind is trying to master the waking confusion resulting from our damaged brain and our high level of emotions. But our memory for what has really happened is so poor that it is so difficult to recall what is dream and what is not. If we get up during the night, and are caught still in this twilight world, we become disoriented and distressed.

Some of us find animals – real or stuffed – help us to visualise concepts such as peace, hope, faith, comfort. Touching their reality can soothe us in this struggle for sleep, as well as in the struggle to know we are awake. My cat is a constant source of comfort during the night, when I wake up frequently and wonder where I am. Her warm, furry and purring body, lying alongside mine under the covers, responds with a little stretch and a small sound whenever I wake up and reach out to touch her during the night. Then I hear the gentle breathing of

Paul beside me, and it reassures me and comforts me, reorienting me to the reality of my bed.

But a stuffed animal can cause alarm! We can mistake what we see so easily. It's like lots of pixels being missing, so we try to make up a picture from a blurred image. My DASNI friend Morris told me that he was out shopping one day, but had to muffle a scream as he walked to the check out. There was a dead cat in his shopping trolley! But as he tried to calm down, and focus more on this terrible sight, he slowly began to realise that it was his own fur hat that he had taken off half an hour before, when he started to do his shopping. Our brains try to make sense of what we see, but it is not always real.

I have seen little stuffed puppies that are very life-like, which have a mechanism inside them like a warm beating heart. I have sat talking to Michelle in her office at the Alzheimer's Association stroking one of these, feeling calmer by the moment. I would love to have one of these later in my journey, when my 'dementia cat' can no longer minister to my needs. But perhaps battery-driven mechanisms could be a problem. I heard that in Japan, when dolls with battery-operated hearts were trialled, former midwives at the nursing home became very distressed when the battery stopped working. Their 'baby' had died, its heart no longer could be felt. So if I do have a 'beating-heart puppy', please check the battery regularly to make sure it is still 'alive'.

These midwives were lucky to have someone able to interpret their apparent delusion, their paranoia, and stress reaction. But such paranoia and delusions are a natural part of us trying to make sense of an increasingly confusing and stressful environment. We create our own stories to explain what is happening. We become non-diplomatic, focused on our own firmly held beliefs as to what is happening around us.

As Victor Frankl, a Holocaust survivor, has said, 'an abnormal reaction to an abnormal situation is normal behaviour.'[43] For people with dementia our behaviour is normal, considering what is happening inside our heads. Try to enter our distorted reality, because if you make us fit in with your reality, it will cause us extra stress. You need to enter into our reality, connect with us by touch, or by look. You need to be authentically present, not far away. You need to realise that we are not far away or lost, but trapped by an inability to communicate and to think clearly, to express this strange mixed-up world being created by our brain damage. Think about this inner reality that we are experiencing, and try to connect with it. Be imaginative, be creative, try to step across the divide between our worlds.

I was visiting a dementia unit in a nursing home, and used to chat with Maureen (not her real name). She could not express herself in any language I could understand, but had created a way of talking that others called 'gibberish'. For her, it was a way to speak out sounds, to express thoughts, fears and feelings. One day, when I went to visit, Maureen was clearly very agitated, and she took me over to the walls near the kitchen area. She pointed out, low to the ground, lots of things, moving – they seemed to be all over the place for her. I said, 'Are there lots of mice here?' Her face beamed. 'Yes!', she was saying to me, by her 'words' – her facial expression and her gestures. As we walked along the corridor, it was clear that there were mice everywhere. Of course, I could not see them, but that did not make them any less real to her.

So I said, 'Let's look for the cat, there must be one around here. Surely the cat will chase away all these mice.' Then we walked around for a while, until excitedly Maureen grabbed my arm and pointed. By her face and the way she made sounds, I could tell she had seen it. There was the cat! And soon she had calmed down, the cat and the mice left her world, and she was able to settle back into the routine of the day.

It is so important to enter into our reality, which is created through scrambled emotion and little cognition, and held together through our spirit, our true self. Our reality may well reflect our emotions, and may tell you something about our worries or our joys, so that you can help us move forward from an unpleasant space, or help us reflect on a happy moment.

Of course, this entering into our reality is far easier to do for those who have some greater emotional distance from us. For our close family members, it is so hard to observe what appears to be a greatly distorted reality, and to react by focusing on the needs of the person with dementia, rather than their own needs in this intimate relationship. This needs to be recognised and to be respected. Professional care workers can do a great deal to relieve our distress, as well as that of our families, by helping in this area of need.

Care-partner, not martyr

Adopting a sole identity as our care-giver highlights our illness and strips both of us of other identities, we have become care-giver and sufferer, in a relationship of co-dependence. You need us to be sick so that you retain your identity as care-giver, otherwise you might feel threatened if we become empowered in any other role.

In this role, you may feel soon overwhelmed by the multitude of tasks, of remembering for two, of planning and organising for two, of covering up our deficits, and grieving over our losses, rather than looking for what remains. You can quickly become exhausted, sad, depressed and in despair. We know how hard it is for you, and we treasure all that you do for us, and know how helpless we have become, but we want the best for you too.

At the same time, if we adopt a sole identity as a sufferer of our illness, we learn helplessness. We lose more function, and show an excess disability, where more dementia is apparent than you might expect from the amount of brain damage we have. This will only add to your burdens as a care-giver, and exacerbate the problem for both of us. It will be a downward spiral to disaster. In this situation, we have become co-dependent, needing each other to accept our labels as victim and sufferer for our identities.

Alternatively, we might cover up our deficits and try to act as if we are normal. This too is a form of co-dependency, because we have put your assumed need ahead of our honest self expression. We want to stop you worrying, to stop this downward spiral, and we pretend at normalcy. But as the disease progresses, we can't keep up this pretence, because it becomes impossible and exhausting, and we become passive and dependent. Suddenly you are faced with the burden we had tried so hard to hold away from you, alone.

Co-dependency is unhealthy for both the person with dementia and their family. We can become more incapable than we really are, and you can become much more exhausted than you need to be. And neither of us is being honest, each of us is journeying alone with dementia, struggling without any true insight as to what to do.

We need to move away from labelling ourselves as care-giver and sufferer, towards becoming a care-partnership, in which we accept, collaborate and adapt to new roles within the journey of dementia. I can become a survivor, a person with dementia, and you can be my care-partner on this journey. I can be a care-partner with you, communicating my true feelings, my true needs, so that you can walk alongside me adjusting and compensating for these expressed needs as we face this struggle together. In this care-partnership, the person with dementia is at the centre of the relationship, not alone as an object to be looked at, as merely a care-recipient. Instead we become an active partner in a circle of care.

Care-partners – family, friends, professionals and governments – should actively seek to understand the person's needs, take full account of existing capabilities, and adjust care levels according to those needs. Listen to us as we try to express these needs and abilities. That way we can dance in celebration together and embrace our shared future.

Spirituality

In the face of declining cognition, and increasing emotional sensitivity, spirituality can flourish as an important source of identity. And yet the stigma that surrounds dementia may lead to restrictions on our ability to develop our spirituality. It threatens our spiritual identity. As time passes, I will need others to understand me, to understand that my odd behaviour, my lack of social graces, my lack of resources to offer in friendship, do not stem from the soul that lies within me. Rather they are simply the product of my diseased brain.

But it is sometimes assumed that our confusion, our lack of speech, and apparent lack of understanding, place us beyond reach of normal spiritual practices, of visiting shrines, worshipping alongside you, and being in communion with God and with others. But to what extent are these assumptions due to the limits placed upon us due to the stigma of our dementia?

You can help us rediscover a sense of meaning in our lives, by finding out what type of activities help us to see beyond the transient worldly difficulties of coping each day with brain damage. By practising our spirituality, we may be able to achieve an identity reflected in the divine, to find emotional security and to discover a real hope in a new future.

Liz MacKinlay has described what she calls the six spiritual tasks of aging, which are equally relevant in dementia: to search for ultimate meaning in life, to respond to that meaning, to move towards final meanings, to find hope, to find intimacy with God and/or others, and to transcend difficulties and losses.[44]

It is important that you find out what our own spiritual tradition has been, and to help us to reconnect with the rituals, the stories, the places, the practices. As a relatively recent Christian, I am not as familiar with the old hymns, but love the new choruses, and more contemporary church worship. I would feel very uncomfortable at a very traditional Christian service, or in another type of religious setting. We need familiar words, tunes, languages and ritual – but ones that are familiar to us, not necessarily to you.

But spirituality is not merely religion. Spirituality is what gives us a sense of meaning and purpose in life, and this may well come from art, nature or music. For me, I treasure nature, I love cats, and I delight in watching all animals in this beautiful creation. It is vital to find out more about the unique individual who has dementia, about their preferences, and then find ways in which this person can be spiritually nourished.

Minister to our true self, which lies beyond cognition and emotion. Perhaps we can be encouraged to write about ourselves. Certainly for me writing my first book was a very important journey of self reflection. When I visited a day care centre in Matsue, I heard some wonderful stories from people about living with dementia, which expressed their true inner feelings and hopes. I could see by their faces what it had meant to them to be helped to write these personal stories.

There are many ways to help us find meaning in our lives. We can be comforted by doll therapy, and I have seen many photos of sheer joy on people's faces – men and women – as they hold their doll. We can be inspired by art or music therapy. We need you to reassure us and to be with us as a guide, as you reach into our spirituality and find ways for us to connect with the divine. Maybe you could use pictures, objects, songs, rituals, activities, places.

Dementia has often been associated with a 'loss of self' and this implies the person travelling the journey with dementia at some stage loses what it is to be human. This is clearly silly, as at what stage can you deny me my selfhood and my spirituality? Exactly when do I cease being me?

I gave a talk at a conference a few years ago, and Liz MacKinlay later edited the paper as a chapter in a book.[45] I said, 'Is cognition the only measure of our presence amongst you as spiritual beings? Certainly my capacity for accurate communication of thought is diminishing daily. It is difficult to find the words for the pictures in my head so as to communicate with you. Does this mean my mind is absent?'

I asked, 'Even if these pictures may one day themselves fade, is my soul connected with this failing cognition?... As I lose an identity in the world around me, which is so anxious to define me by what I do and say rather than who I am, I can seek an identity by simply being me, a person created in the image of God. My spiritual self is reflected in the divine and given meaning as a transcendent being.'

I am daily losing more and more bits of my temporal lobe, yet I have read that electrical stimulation of the temporal lobe gives intense spiritual experiences. Does this mean my God-experience will in some way fade, and my spirituality will disappear? Surely not! I am much more than a diseased brain.

In my talk I said, 'My creation in the divine image is as a soul capable of love, sacrifice and hope, not as a perfect human being, in mind or body. I want you to relate to me in that way, seeing me as God sees me.'

Will I know God if I can no longer remember? In my first book[46] I wrote 'As I unfold before God, as this disease unwraps me, opens up the treasures of what lies within my multi-fold personality, I can feel safe as each layer is gently opened out. God's everlasting arms will be beneath me, upholding me.' As we people with dementia lose our memory of who we are, we become reflected in others. In the family of God, the body of Christ, I am what others remember of me.

I need you to relate directly to my spirit, and as I travel this journey of dementia, I will rely on others increasingly to support my spirituality.[47] There is no stage in this journey at which you must abandon all hope of connecting with me, as we can remain linked through our spirits – not our minds. You can minister to my spirit in song, prayer, ritual, and by your spiritual presence alongside me.

You play a vital role in relating to the soul within me, connecting at this eternal level. Sing alongside me, touch me, pray with me, reassure me of your presence, and through you of Christ's presence. Be creative and trust in God to help you bring his love to me. Identify where I find meaning in life, to discover and enrich my spirituality. Through this I can find spiritual healing and transcend my sense of loss and fear.

For you to connect with us spirit to spirit at this level requires sensitivity to what gives us sense of meaning, what faith tradition, what ritual, what worship practice. Focus on the reality of the present, the simple joy of creation. You can reach across cultures, across faiths, by touching our spirit in ritual, nature, song, music, dance, or other ways to connect us with the ground of all being, the divine.

4

I Know Who I'll Be When I Die

An identity crisis!

The dementia script – the shock of diagnosis and horror of prognosis – is a turning point in our lives. That moment is etched in our memories. What the weather was like, what people were wearing, and what people said emerge from the fog of our distorted memories as one clear crystal picture. For some of us it is a relief. At last there is an explanation for our confusion, slowness, memory loss and daily difficulties. But we must still face up to what the future now holds. For others diagnosis leads to disbelief. There is nothing wrong with us, surely! No one can think we are anything like those people in nursing homes, who don't know who they are or who their families are?

And for others, like me, it is a time of trauma. I faced an awful awareness of my future, of what lay ahead for me and for my girls. I would have to stop work, and would still need to support the family. My world had collapsed. Everything had changed. I faced a defeat of spirit and of hope.

Our main fear is the 'loss of self' associated with dementia. We face an identity crisis. We all believe the toxic lie of dementia that the mind is absent and the body is an empty shell. Our sense of self is shattered with this new label of dementia. Who am I, if I can no longer be a valued member of society? What if I don't know my family, if I don't know who I am and who I was, if I don't even know God?

Our first thoughts after diagnosis often turn to who we are and who we will become. We face an identity crisis. We have a fear of the future, a fear of decline, and a fear of death in a state of unknowing. We can no longer be defined by our work, our contribution to the community, but have a new identity thrust upon us as a diseased person – no longer valued by society, no longer needed for making any contribution. Suddenly we have become a non-person.

The day before my diagnosis I was a busy and successful single mother with three girls, and a high-level executive job with the Australian Government. The day after I was a label – Person with Dementia. No one knew what to say, what to expect of me, how to talk to me, even whether to visit me. I had become a labelled person, defined by my disease overnight. It was like I had a target painted on my forehead, shouting out for all the world to see that I was blind-folded, no longer able to function in society.

But we can find a new identity as an emotional being. We can hug, we can have cuddly toys once more, we can cry and express pain more freely. In our relationships, we can connect at a deeper level. We have inner psychic resources that arise from our personality and life story. These resources – our attitude – affect how we cope with brain damage. For some of us, of course, our life story offers us no resilience, no help in tackling this latest battle for existence. Our resources are minimal, and we have little to draw on. But if we give up, we appear to have a greater degree of dementia.

Importantly, even beyond our psyche, our emotional and psychological reactions forged in the crucible of life, each of us has a spiritual self. Even without words for the pictures in our mind, and without being able to draw on some sort of inner strength, we can find meaning in life in our own spirituality. This is where you can minister to us, connect with us and empower us. My Christian faith, my spiritual relationship with God through Jesus, certainly strengthened as an important source of my identity, despite the fear of ceasing to be.

It is what lies right at our spiritual core that is truly important, and this can be ministered to with sensitivity to what is giving us meaning in our lives with dementia. 'It is only with the heart that one can see rightly; what is essential is invisible to the eye.'[48] With this phrase, Antoine de Saint Exupéry expressed the importance of our inner self, our spirit self.

The fear of ceasing to be

During my first two years of living a life transformed by this label of dementia, I felt shame and retreated from society. I had a terrible fear about my future, how would it feel to die with this disease? I was encouraged to write about these feelings, and wrote my first book. My biggest fear was the later stages when I will not know who I am, who my family and friends are, and maybe even not know God.

We face this awful fear of ceasing to be. It's not just a physical death that we face, but also a gradual emotional and psychological death. It's journey into ceasing to be. In some ways you can prepare yourself for death, knowing who you are and how you will be likely to cope with this. But with dementia it is so different. I was terrified that I wouldn't know who I was, who anybody was, that I would be totally lost and not able to cope with death. And this fear is set in the midst of a struggle to retain a sense of who we are now, let alone who we were, or who we are becoming.

Fear can transform us into deniers, when we pretend we are well and nothing is wrong. The fragile shell of normalcy protects us from our fears. And our family and friends deny there is a problem, as a defence against their own feelings of grief and anger. Or we can become victims, collapsing into a paralysis of fear, giving up our willingness to keep trying to function. And our family and friends adopt the new identity of care-givers, smothering us with their concerns and taking over our daily lives.

But we can find a better way of reacting with realism to the diagnosis, by reflecting on the totality of who we are. We are far more than a cognitive self. We are emotional beings with relationships in this world with others. We are spiritual selves in relationship with the divine. Martin Buber writes, 'Through the Thou a person becomes I.'[49] Through the centering of my life, by focusing on my spirit in relationship with the divine, I am becoming who I really am.

The challenge is to draw on our psychic resources to step across that yawning chasm of fear that opened up at that moment of diagnosis. How can we live in a world of hope, alternatives, growth and possibility, when dementia threatens our sense of self?

We need to create a new image of who we are and who we are becoming. How we do this depends very much on our personality, our life story, our health, our spirituality, and our social environment. We can choose the attitude we have, and some of us, like Frankl, can try to look for meaning in our lives through the attitude we take toward unavoidable suffering.

It has been a long journey for me since 1995 to learn how to live positively each day with my diagnosis of dementia, when I questioned who I will be when I die with dementia. Now I realise that I will still be me, my eternal self which is my spirit. My spirit is me and will always be me. Even through the ravages of dementia, my spirit will remain intact and continue to be the primary way in which God works within me. I can survive this disease with dignity, confident that God sees my spirit – the true me. My spirit remains my mainstay, as I travel this path of making meaning in life, and of discovering the glory of God within me.

Who am I becoming?
The journey of self discovery
My journey with dementia has been a journey of self discovery about who I really am. My first book asked 'Who will I be when I die?' It expressed the fear of ceasing to be, and assumed that the journey of dementia was somehow a loss of self. But over the last few years, I have

done a lot of thinking about what makes up a person, and what is happening to us as we journey into dementia. Dementia is often thought of as death by small steps, but we must ask ourselves what is really dying. Hasn't the person with dementia reached that place of 'now', of existing actively in the present?

I believe that people with dementia are making an important journey from cognition, through emotion, into spirit. I've begun to realise what really remains throughout this journey is what is really important, and what disappears is what is not important. I think that if society could appreciate this, then people with dementia would be respected and treasured.

There is the cognitive outer self, which is the self – the mask – that we are presenting, when we are at work or at home. Organising, planning, writing, speaking, shopping, cooking, all sorts of complex activities make up what we think is who we are. We have labels for ourselves, names, jobs, addresses, memories about our past, ideas for our future. We communicate these as part of defining our outer masks. When we meet each other, it is a description of our masks that we seek when we say, 'What is your name, where do you live, what do you do?'

But there is another layer just beneath, an emotional layer, that defines the way we relate to others. That is the mask that I use when I relate to Paul and to my daughters, or speak to my friends and family. And that is how I show my feelings. This emotional layer is becoming more and more scrambled in our journey with dementia. It is less predictable, we are less in control, and our feelings are more disjointed.

Beneath this increasingly jumbled layer of emotion is the true self that remains intact despite the ravages of dementia. This is my spiritual self or transcendent self. It is the 'me' that relates to the beauty of a garden, of the leaves or the flowers; it is the 'me' that relates to God; it is my spirit, the essence of me.

This real self cannot exist independently in our society, which defines people by the outer layers of cognition and emotion, by our masks. I couldn't survive in society without Paul, despite living an authentic life in the present, as a spiritual self, because today's society expects you to function like a 'normal' person, with a past, memories, and a knowledge of what day it is and what you should have done, what you did yesterday and what you are going to do tomorrow.

My spiritual self exists in the 'now', with no past or future. The Buddhist word *setsuna* captures this sense of existence independent of time. We can more fully appreciate the divine, which is outside of time, as the 'now' which is the ground of all being.[50]

Living in the present is where our true self is. If we get too anxious about what might happen or what used to happen, we are really in our outer shell of ourselves, and that's not really us. I've come to the acceptance of living in the present, and realising that it is a very special privilege to be released from memories and future worries.

Like a bud, my true self encapsulates all the potential of what it means to be me, in an eternal realm, not only in this earthly temporal existence. This being in the present, continually and eternally, is a new way of living, maybe even the essence of living.

Zen mind is ordinary mind

A meditation written by Morris from DASNI captures this essence of living:

> The rain had washed clean the air, and the sky was now filled with fluffy clouds. Walking along the gravel road I watched three deer, two big ones and a little one, gracefully climb the sunlit hill and disappear over the top. I thought about meditation. I remembered how, before Alzheimer's, I used to think about meditation from time to time.
>
> Zen Buddhism pointed out that the mind was like a chattering monkey swinging from branch to branch, from anxious thought to greedy thought. How much quality of experience could one have with a mind like that? The path of meditation offered to silence the mind, making it like a still mountain pool reflecting the moonlight. With such a mind one could savor the ecstasy of Now. That was an interesting idea.
>
> My monkey mind went south three years ago. This would perhaps be a great advantage for meditation, except that my ability to concentrate has gone as well. I can no longer hope to

cultivate mindfulness until, with lightning discernment, I can instantly perceive the Illusion at the core of grasping thoughts and, like a samurai laser swordsman, vaporize them into Emptiness. In a couple of years I'll be lucky to have enough mindfulness to cook a frozen dinner in the microwave.

So when I looked at the deer, I thought, 'I'll never see them any better.' But, strangely, this thought was not depressing. I sensed that images of the silent mind had ceased to grasp me, and having abandoned hope of the ecstasy of Now, I understood what the Zen Masters were trying to get at. Zen mind is Ordinary mind.[51]

I'm becoming who I really am!

As we journey towards our spiritual self, as our outer masks decrease, our inner self increases. Cognition is fading, emotion and spirit are increasing. We can be strengthened in our spirit as we make this journey with dementia.

My DASNI friend, Shirl Garnett from Australia, said recently in an email to me,

> I think the most releasing realisation I came to early in my journey with dementia was that, the further I progressed with the physical/psychological decline the more my spirit man increased in proportion. My relationship with the Lord, while good before, has become even closer and I know that, no matter how far I go in this journey I will retain my relationship Spirit to spirit.[52]

She wants people to 'realise how important that spiritual relationship is in navigating the waters we find ourselves in.'[53]

I have learned to trust in God, and to watch in amazement as he unfolds my life before me, as I take each step in faith. I find the Berber saying that 'Life is a loom on which God holds the threads' speaks to me, as I let God work in my life.[54] By walking in trust each day, an amazing tapestry of life is being laid out before me, and as I look over my shoulder I can see a beautiful picture emerging, a meaning for my existence and a purpose for my life.

Since writing my first book, and grappling with the fear of ceasing to be, I have worked through what it means to be 'me', and have been able to answer the question it posed. I realise what it is that I am losing, and what will always remain. I now know that in this journey towards my true self, with dementia stripping away the layers of cognition and emotion, I'm becoming who I really am.

It's a totally different way of thinking from when I was first diagnosed, when I started my journey with dementia. I am no longer the outer layer, the outer mask, of who I used to be, which was the working mother of three daughters, the family concerns, home life and work issues. Instead, I am revealing more of the inner person. This person existed back then, but she was obscured by the masks of achieved cognition and controlled emotion.

I am more emotional now. Before becoming ill, I was always calm, cool and controlled as well as controlling. I never really connected with people at the level of their feelings. I was task-oriented, with my emotions restricted to my daughters. Now my emotions are more open, and I have more concern for people's feelings. I relate more to the whole person, rather than simply the outer mask.

It is interesting to read Viktor Frankl describe the psychological journey made by survivors of the trauma of Auschwitz.[55] From illusion, denial and anger as first responses, through to apathy and humour as defences, people eventually found inner peace in the spirituality of religion, art and music. For people struggling with the journey of dementia, it is a similar path of survival, of illusion, denial, anger, apathy, humour and a search for meaning. We are following a path of suffering to find the inner person, the true spirit self. In the prison camp of dementia, in the trials of our daily struggle and the horror of what is to come, we can find meaning in suffering.

What we find is that each one of us can say, 'I am who I am, not what I say or do'. Who I am is defined by my spirit. In life, cognition and emotion may change, but our spirit is our essence, held in the grip of the divine. Our spirit was known before we were in our mother's womb, and will be known long after we have become dust. It is a journey into simplicity, one that moves away from the outer mask of cognition. This is the façade we present to the world, of what we do, where we work or live, how we speak and the ideas and views we communicate in words to others.

The next layer of this complex self is emotions. Here lie our feelings, our love for others, our hurts and hopes, our relationships. This becomes increasingly scrambled in the journey of dementia, as we experience emotions in an unpredictable way.

At the centre of our being lies the true self, what identifies us to be truly human, truly unique, and truly the person we were born to be. This is our spiritual heart, the centre from which we draw meaning in this rush from birth to death, whenever we pause long enough to look beyond our cognition, through our clouded emotions into what lies within.

For the person with dementia, this is what remains intact, it is what makes us who we really are. One day my body will be in the foetal position, curled up, unaware of my surroundings, barely able to function, but my spiritual self will live on, my spiritual connection with this body will be stepping away into a new life. Heaven is where I'm headed.

Dancing with dementia

My journey into the spirit is freeing, but I am still living in a cognitive world. Daily life is a struggle. It would be easier just to be. But I am surviving this journey with dementia and, rather than fighting the disability, I am adapting to it in a dance. As each decline becomes apparent, I let Paul know, and together as a care-partnership, we work out a way to change our behaviour.

The situation is changing every few months, something that is different in the way we manage our lives, just little things, but noticeable. We adjust to change, in the dance with dementia, which has new music being played all the time as I decline and communicate my needs. Paul needs to make a new dance step, I make a new step, we follow or lead, and it is a compromise. The dance of dementia is not an easy one, because dementia in many ways is a disease of society, where the person and their family is isolated by stigma. It's not much fun.

My family was shattered by the trauma of my dementia, but now in this journey I think we are discovering new dimensions of each other. Maybe we are rising like a phoenix out of the ashes of that terrible time, and I think we are all more mature as a result. In a special way, Paul as a care-partner has come into this dance much later, and chosen to make this journey alongside me and my daughters. He does not have the pain of the past to deal with, the grief of losses and the continual comparison of the person I am now, to the person I seemed to be before diagnosis.

For my daughters, it is a more difficult dance, which they did not choose to join, but were forced to participate in. They have losses to grieve over, and issues to deal with. Their future is changed now, and they must adapt to the idea of a mother who is losing cognition and becoming more scrambled emotionally each day. They must also address their fear of what happens later, in the end stage, when little remains except my spirit self. But in the dance of dementia, I hope that they too will find the connection with me, spirit to spirit, and be able to hear the music of change, and adapt to me becoming who I really am.

I'm choosing an attitude of dancing with dementia. I'm choosing to be a survivor. I'm choosing to live my life positively everyday. I love the imagery of a couple dancing with dementia. It's a couple, a care-partnership, in which we move together. We sense each other's needs, and change and adapt according to the changing music of the journey with dementia. It's a very expressive way, I think, talking about the care partnership being like a dance with dementia. This dance image might help to see what is going on, to us and around us. On diagnosis, our care network – family members, friends, community links, professionals and workplace – may react by either denying the practical realities of the diagnosis or by assuming the role of over-whelming care-giver – you must do everything because we can't do anything.

In the denying reaction, needs are not assessed, and as behaviour patterns change, the changes, perceived as losses, become the focus of attention. In the overwhelming care-giver reaction, your emphasis on loss undermines our self esteem, creates unnecessary stresses across the care network and contributes to a downward spiral of helplessness in us.

As our care-partner, do you try to do what you have always done, or do you learn new steps, sense the movements to trust one another? The overwhelming care-giver immediately takes over all of our functions, smothering us with love and attention, thereby discounting remaining capabilities, undermining our self-esteem and placing focus on the care-giver identity in the relationship.

But like all dance partners, as care-partners in the dance with dementia, we both have to learn to *listen* to the music. What is happening to me, to us? What is the rhythm of our dance with dementia? Is it fast or slow? Who is in charge?

The care-partner asks: 'What do you want?'; 'What can I do to help?'; importantly, 'What can you do, or what would you like to be helped to do?' The phrase 'use it or lose it' is important, and it does not matter how small the function, it is still important to retain as much as possible. We dance together, each of us adjusting our steps as we adjust to each new challenge of dementia.

And we need to watch the musicians – the care network. Professionals, family, friends provide cues and support for our dance with dementia. And they should be watching us dance, not playing their own music! If you are a musician in the care network, then you too need to watch the dance floor carefully, maybe adjust your rhythm to ours, maybe play a different tune. You too are part of this dance with dementia!

But like all dances, there will be times when one partner is in charge, times when partners are separate, and times when the lead changes. Questions you might be asking as you, our care-partner, watch how we are coping with the dance steps of dementia include: 'Do you want to drive? Do you want to cook? Do you want to do the washing? Do you want to do the shopping? Can you manage the shower? What about the telephone? Can you eat OK? What about your medication? What about daily planning?'

Or are our diminishing energy and resources better spent on being with our family, writing, talking to others, caring for the garden, praying, walking, reading, looking after the animals? You know we can't do as much, so let's both adjust the dance so that we do what is important, meaningful and sustaining to us, and through us to you.

By accepting this journey of change and adaptation, we can dance with dementia and choose a new life in the slow lane.

Choosing to dance

It has been a long journey now, of knowing I have this death sentence, this dementia, hanging over me. Time to grieve, time to focus on what I am losing, but also time to celebrate life each day, smell the flowers, and focus on what will stay with me forever. God will always be there, Paul and my girls will always surround me with love, and I will be part of a beautiful creation, moving along with it, enjoying the moments as they go by.

Of course we desperately seek and hope for a cure, but in the meantime, we struggle to remain as well as possible for as long as possible. We can find out how much music we can still make with what we have left, as we celebrate this new life in the slow lane. We can find new ways to enjoy each moment of our day. For me it is the beauty of a sunset, of seeing my daughters' joys and triumphs, of stroking cats and hugging my husband.

As we dance with dementia, to struggle to cope, we can still create and dazzle, despite our limitations. We can develop new talents, the pearls hidden within us, by focusing on relationships and on greater emotional and spiritual connection, rather than on cognition. By assigning cognition a secondary place, being content with our new life, we can enhance these other aspects of our personality. We can rediscover our spirituality, developing a greater awareness of what gives us meaning in life. My Christian faith certainly flourished, as I turned to God in anger, fear, confusion, and eventually acceptance.

We cannot change our illness, but we can change our attitude to it. This is enough to transform our life. All of us can choose our attitude each day. I choose to be a survivor. In describing life in Auschwitz, Viktor Frankl said, 'Any man can, even under such circumstances, decide what shall become of him, mentally and spiritually.'[56] And for the person with dementia, our circumstances mean that our care-partner can play an important role in helping us to make the choices that free us, that give us inner freedom and allow us to retain our human dignity.

A Buddhist saying captures the importance of choosing our attitude: 'View the world from a different perspective, the world is vast and wide. Change to a different viewpoint in your relationships and in dealing with all matters, everything will be light and easy.'

For me, dementia is a gift – precious time to account for life, to reflect on my eternal spirit and its relationships with the divine, to reflect before God. Psalm 23 of the Bible reassures me with these words: 'Even though I walk through the valley of the shadow of death, I will fear no evil, for you are with me.'

It is through finding meaning in life, even in dementia, that we can create a new sense of becoming, and overcome our fear of loss. By working through our fear, we can begin to feel joy. We are on a path to healing, through feeling and acknowledging our fear, anxiety, and the ebbs and flows of confusion.

By casting aside the lie of dementia, that we are losing our selfhood, we can work towards creating a new future, of being a survivor. Our passage towards this choice will be a struggle of feeling to achieve healing. Most importantly, on this journey, we can come to realise that we are uniquely qualified to reach out to you, our families and friends walking alongside us on this journey with dementia.

And many of us find self validation in giving of ourselves to others. I find this expressed in a Buddhist saying: 'Give without expectation and give with gratitude, for giving will reap the greatest harvest.' As a Christian, I am called to help others, to love others as Jesus loves them, as if I could see the world from their eyes, and knew all of their pains and joys. To reach out to others, and to seek inner healing, will take great determination. Determination is about getting back into the driving seat of life. We are confronting the fear of a living death, drawing on our inner resources. We can overcome our feelings of inertia, of exhaustion, as we face this journey of dementia with courage.

We need to find the pearl hidden within us. Like the pearl that is formed through the irritation of a grain of sand within an oyster, our pearl has formed through the challenge of living with dementia. Finding this pearl within is the key to creating a new future of life in the slow lane.

To cope in this confusing reality is a struggle. My keys for coping are a strong Christian faith, the love of friends and family, anti-dementia drugs, and a positive attitude. Our faith, or our spirituality, is crucial. We are losing our cognitive self – even a reliable and coherent emotional self. What remains is our spirituality. We need you to help us connect with our faith – to whatever has given us true meaning in life. The meaning I choose is an attitude, of love for others, of love for the creator, and of acceptance of a meaning in my disease. It is not what we want from life but what we give to it! This is our purpose, and dementia is a journey in which we can explore this meaning and connect with others.

My Christian faith has helped me to find a meaning even in suffering. It gives me hope, and helps me to avoid the self-pity that leads to depression, and gives me a focus on helping others. It is helping me to accept that I am still really very much me, and that I still have a relationship with other people, and with God.

I treasure every single moment of life and realise that my time on this earth is not what's most important. Although I'll do what I can while I'm here, my action is not what is most important to me. It is rather my eternal life that is important, and that remains in my spirit through and beyond this journey with dementia. My faith gives me a different perspective. And with those different glasses on, as it were, it enables me to cope so much better.

Now, even with dementia, I can live without despair and unhelpful self-pity, relying on God's unconditional love. I do not need to do anything to earn it except to be me, even as I am with dementia. We are all accepted as wonderful and whole human beings. God values each one of us, and we need to see ourselves as God sees us – as a very special person of great value and worth. My situation has not changed, but I feel so different about it.

The love of family and friends surrounds us and gives security, an oasis of emotional warmth in an otherwise confusing world. You are our care-partners on this journey, and we need you to understand us, and to meet our needs as we become less and less able to deal with this illness. The care-partner can be the husband or wife, the daughter or son, the staff at the day care centre, the Alzheimer's Association, or any other person in a helping relationship with the person with dementia. You give us hope and encouragement, and help us to overcome our deficits in a positive way.

The love of my family and friends – most importantly Paul and my daughters – helps me through each day, and gives me the security and hope that I need for the future. I have lots of deficits, but Paul compensates for these, adjusting his every response as my care-partner so that I can function to the best of my ability. In living this dance with dementia, my care-partner and I take steps that match each other. His steps guide me round this dance floor of life.

Drugs or complementary medication are important to clear the fog. They give me the ability to speak, and to remain aware of and concerned about what is happening around me. Without them, I am apathetic, unable to cope with daily life. I would be no longer able to speak, think or do much at all. I would still have faith and hope, be surrounded in love, but be unable to communicate clearly, to enjoy living, to be able to do as much as possible for myself for as long as possible.

My attitude has transformed the pattern of my life, and I choose to live positively with dementia, drawing on my inner psychic resources and my spirituality to view each day, each hour, as a gift. We can all choose how we will react to a new life. So our first step is to find out what we can celebrate. We can choose to find joy in being sensitive in our relationships, in being more open to our spirituality, and in finding positive aspects of living in the slow lane. For me the first steps to celebrate were retiring from work and being able to pick up my daughters after school in the light, rather than race home to see them in the dark after a long day at work.

I choose a new identity as a survivor. I want to learn to dance with dementia. I want to live positively each day, in a vital relationship of trust with my care-partners alongside me. By rejecting the lie of dementia, and focusing on my spirit rather than my mind, I can be free of fear of loss of self, and in so doing can also help you to lose your fear that you are losing me.

I look towards new horizons of hope, as we people with dementia seek liberation from internalising the oppressor of dementia. To live with 'the fear of ceasing to be' takes enormous courage. The precious string of pearls, of memories, that is our life, is breaking, the pearls are being lost. But by finding new pearls, those created in the struggle with dementia, we can put together a new necklace of life, of hope in our future.

Each person with dementia is as worthy and precious as a beautiful newborn baby, a gift for us all to cherish. With our damaged brain, we have no memory of how you might have hurt us in the past, no worries about what you might do to us in the future, and no idea what we might have done to, or neglected to do for you. All we can do is intensely experience the 'now' of each moment with you. Treasure these moments and you will be able to share true acceptance of self.

We need to express our voices together, from our different perspectives, of this interdependent struggle to live with the unpredictability and irrationality of dementia. Each person with dementia is a gift, and has a great deal of wisdom about life. It is those around us who need to unwrap this beautiful package.

We seek a new paradigm of dementia survival with dignity, walking with you on that journey from diagnosis to death. This journey of survival, of uncovering the inner spirit, is a journey of letting go, and finding inner peace, as expressed in the Buddhist saying: 'A wise person is able to let go. To let go is actually to receive boundless happiness.' For me, my journey has taken me into an ever deeper and more trusting relationship with God, knowing he loves me just as I am, my true inner self. I have been able to 'Let go and let God'.

As survivors of the journey with dementia, we can share with you the insider's knowledge that we have. We are confronting a living death, and we are trying to find ways to liberate ourselves from this fear of ceasing to be. We know what it was once like to be normal, like you. We know both your world and ours. We have stepped into this new world of dementia. It is as if we are bi-cultural, and have stepped across the divide between your world and ours.

With your understanding and support, we can help you to help us. We can make history together. Find a way to listen to our broken voices, our disjointed thoughts, and our fragmented memories of how things are and used to be. Let's work together to share our insights as equal partners – people with dementia, their families, and those who support them – on this journey from diagnosis to death.

Afterword

D ear reader, I thank you for letting me share my journey with you. Much has changed since I stumbled onto the dementia dance floor. There is medication, there is better understanding, there is better support. But there is still no cure, and much remains to be done to break down barriers of stigma and ignorance about this disease.

There were many times when I despaired of ever finishing this book. It has been a real effort to get my thoughts together. I have given my best. If you have dementia, I hope that some of what I have written may help you feel less alone. If you are a care-partner, I hope you might understand us a little better.

It has been a tremendous struggle to collect together all my thoughts, talks, speeches, correspondence, notes and so on, for the last six years. Inspiration, rather than memory, has been the thread that enabled me to weave these disjointed fragments into this book.

'The years have gone by yet in many ways yesterday is as tomorrow, real though distant, old as history yet as new as the next sunrise. The memory of writing these words eludes me. Their truth however makes all the struggles and heartaches seem as nothing.'[57]

But I am tired and I need to turn my computer off. I am feeling burnt-out, exhausted, no longer able to make this type of sustained effort any more. It is time to move away from the bright lights to a corner of the floor where the rhythm is slower and the music quieter, but still sweet. All I can do now is sit quietly and listen, and hope for a cure.

Beachmere, July 2004

APPENDIX 1

Do You Believe In Miracles?

It was a cold, windy October evening and Paul got a bit lost as we tried to find the venue for my talk to a women's group in Goulburn. I had been invited by the ecumenical church men's group to speak at this dinner, which they had cooked, were serving and organising for their lady folk.

I could barely speak, though, having lost my voice due to a very bad dose of flu, and felt snuffly and a bit shivery. Hardly after-dinner speaker material! So I sat with a group of lovely ladies and tried to make conversation despite the limitations of my voice and the need to frequently blow my nose. I was an uninspiring sight, I am sure! Soon, all too soon, dessert had been served and eaten – by our menfolk all dressed in white shirts, black trousers and bow ties – and I was being introduced. I prayed a silent prayer as I walked to the microphone – I needed to be able to get through this with my voice threatening to give up entirely at any minute.

Where had this started? The previous evening, the phone had rung and my daughter took the call. 'Mum,' she said, 'it's for you.' I took the phone and said 'Hello'. 'Hello, this is Ian.' My mind spun the wheel of fortune, trying to guess who this was. 'Yes?', I said, sort of with a question mark. He must have guessed I was a complete blank. 'Ian Lyon.' Hum. Still no luck with the wheel. It spun round and got no matches.

Even more alarmingly, with my obvious uncertainty, he then said, 'You're our guest speaker for tomorrow night.' Now alarm bells were being set off in my head. Vaguely I remembered being asked to do something like this months ago, but had seen nothing in writing, talked to no one, and had nothing in my trusty memory bank – the diary.

'I think you'd better talk to my husband,' I said, in a complete panic. First of all, I could hardly speak, having a bad dose of flu. Secondly, I would have to write a talk, and Paul would have to drive me there and back, and still get up to catch the early flight to Melbourne on Saturday morning.

But you know what it is like with God, those sorts of things don't really matter to him. After all, with him, all things are possible.

Paul came gleefully back upstairs, and I said, smiling, 'I suppose we're going to Goulburn tomorrow night!' So there we were, in Goulburn on a cold blustery evening! And I started to speak these words.

> Well, I want to tell you a bit about healing – it really happens today, not just 2,000 years ago. And you don't need bucket-loads of faith, or be very holy or important, to be healed.
>
> Nor do you have to be brave – you can be very fearful, like I was, very down at heart, and not believing God could heal me, when I was diagnosed with Alzheimer's Disease five years ago. I was told I would be in a nursing home by the year 2000, and dead a few years after that from this horrific terminal illness.
>
> *Who will I be when I die?*, the title of my first book, expresses my fears about dying with dementia – will I know who I am, who my family and friends are? Most importantly, will I still know God? But here I am, still alive and well, living with considerable brain damage, which if you only looked at my scans would have you booking me into the nearest nursing home. But when you listen and talk to me, this is God at work, our miracle worker. Surely the Holy Spirit is filling those empty spaces in my brain, giving me much joy and peace, as well as helping me to cope with daily life.
>
> Maybe some of us think that good people never got sick, and that sickness comes from some sin in your life. The Bible, in the Old Testament, describes a man called Job, who lost his wealth and his health. His friends said to him he must have done something very wrong for this to have happened. His wife suggested he give up on his God. But Job kept believing in God's goodness, and that somehow God knew much more than him about what this was all about and why he might be suffering. He remained faithful, yet puzzled by his God. I had quite a few letters when I was first diagnosed with Alzheimer's Disease, suggesting that there must be some sin or lack of forgiveness in my life that needed to be dealt with, which upset me. I had enough questions of my own to ask God, without any further uncertainty!
>
> But I do believe that we can be healed, from illnesses of our spirit, our emotion and our physical body. I do believe that I am

being healed, even though I am not as well as I was. I know that spiritually and emotionally there has been huge growth in my life! Sometimes we are not healed in any areas, other times we are. It is all a mystery, just like life is a mystery, as are illness and death, and what lies beyond.

In the Bible, in the New Testament, witnesses have written about Jesus doing acts of healing, and being mobbed by crowds of people wanting to be healed. They report that Jesus told his 12 disciples to cure every disease and every sickness, and gave the same command to 70 people he chose to go out amongst the surrounding villages.

Healing was one of the last things he told his friends about after coming back from the dead, and before finally disappearing from their sight. He said that people who believed in him would lay hands on the sick and they will recover. The first followers of Jesus were evidence of this, and descriptions of their actions talk about crowds gathering to see many who were paralysed or lame being cured.

So if I think we can heal, how do I think we go about it? And does healing still happen today, or did it stop about 2,000 years ago? Is there some special way to pray? Do we have to lay hands on someone? Do we have to be very holy or righteous to pray for healing?

I am no theologian and can only talk to you about my own personal journey with healing over the last five years. But I still have some tough questions about healing, to ask God one day: Why are some healed and others not? Why do we all die eventually of something or other? And what if a blind person came up to you right now and asked you to pray for her healing? You might put your hands on her head, even over her eyes, and maybe pray for healing. But would you really expect it to happen, for her to suddenly be able to see and to race outside to tell her friends and family that God has restored her sight?

When I was told I had Alzheimer's Disease and would decline rapidly into advanced dementia within about five years, I was scared! I realised that the disease eats away at the brain, so that slowly it disappears and you lose all sorts of abilities, like talking, writing, walking, till in the end you slip into a coma and die. There is no cure and there are no stories of remission, unlike cancer.

To believe I could defy dementia was a test of my faith – as well as for everyone in my church who was praying for me. I had struggled with my faith in healing, feeling somehow a bit of a fraud in praying for it, as I really didn't expect it to happen. So I did not pray for my own healing, and just let others do that for me.

But God has done and is still doing amazing things in my life, and has given me much joy and showered me with blessings through all of this. I don't deny I have dementia, and that I am getting sicker each month, each year, but certainly the decline is far slower than expected. I am not sure what each of us thinks is meant by the word 'healing'. I have learned a lot about healing in my journey with dementia. I have come to realise that healing can and does happen, and that it is far more than just the physical cure that we in our simple worldly perspective hope for, but struggle to believe in.

Already the damage to my brain clearly visible in scans is such that I should be much more disabled by now. But my brain is still functioning quite well despite all the missing bits. Is this healing? I believe it is only part of the story – and not the most important part.

Healing is more than just physical healing, we can be healed in two other areas – spiritual and emotional. These are even more important, surely, for our spiritual healing is an eternal solution, not one only for this world. And our emotional healing has so much bearing on all our relationships in this world with God, our family and our friends.

The other problem we seem to have with healing is that we expect it to be instant. But so often we get sick bit by bit, so why not get better physically, emotionally, spiritually – by tiny steps?

For me, healing is wholeness of the body, mind and spirit, where wholeness of the body is the physical healing we all focus on so much, wholeness of the mind is the emotional healing needed to restore us in our relationships, and wholeness of the spirit is the eternal spiritual healing that surpasses all other forms of healing.

I know that I have been healed spiritually and emotionally of the doubt of where God might be in all of this, and of the fear of the disease itself, of the way it takes away the mind bit by bit. But this spiritual and emotional healing happened in stages for me, and I describe some of this in my first book.

All along, too, in my heart I did not believe in my own physical healing, a cure. But I was really challenged to ask for prayer when late in 1996 I started experiencing hallucinations. By 1997 they really scared me and I speak in my first book of how I spent a terrible night, dragging myself to church the next day, weary and burdened with fear, and sought prayer after the service. I had never prayed for my own healing, although lots of other people were praying for me. I thought Alzheimer's was too hard and I couldn't see why God would bother with me – I was no Mother Teresa with a great mission.

I only asked three people to pray, and just for the hallucinations to stop. I set these limits on God, as I doubted in 'real' healing. Closing my eyes, I did not realise a 'prayer scrum' of almost the whole congregation had formed around me. Of course, they did not know about these limits so they all asked for me to get better.

Only later, much later, was I told what had happened. All I knew was that the hallucinations stopped that night, but then also I began to get a bit better and did not understand why. I did not know anyone had asked for more than I had expected.

Over the following weeks my brain was much less foggy. I was able to speak a little better, and not get too many words mixed up or confused. I began to do much more than before, even being able to visit shopping centres and other busy places without getting too exhausted. I started driving my car again.

A month or so before the prayer scrum at church, I had sent the draft manuscript for my book off to some publishers. It was not until I had begun to get better that HarperCollins got back to me saying they wanted to publish it. I said I would have to add a chapter or so on healing, and over the next month or so finished the book. It was almost as if God had waited to heal me, until he was sure I would write about it!

I must admit, though it is hard to get used to the idea that maybe, just maybe, I might be defying this dementia. We had planned on my steady decline, as medically expected. And here God has put a spanner in the works. So we take each day as it comes.

We need to try and believe in my healing – really believe – and to realise that prayers have been zapped up to God from around the world for my healing. Didn't we really expect him to do something as a result? We may well have been faithful in prayer, but have we been faithful in our belief that he will answer us?

I have been and am being healed emotionally and spiritually. I can also say that I am not declining with dementia as fast as expected. But I still struggle with the doubt of a complete cure, even though I am living the experience of a more holistic healing moment by moment.

Unlike cancer, I have never heard of remissions or healing from Alzheimer's disease, so it really will be able to be seen as a miracle, a witness to God's power! But which is greater, a physical cure or my spiritual healing? Is it best to say, 'I am physically healed, praise God', or to say, 'I know all my sins are forgiven, and I go happily and at peace to meet the Lord of my life.'

For me the last statement is greater, because it is an eternal solution, not one that only applies to this short earthly life. I prefer an eternity of forgiveness and being with Jesus, to a transient cure here on earth.

Of course I'd like complete physical healing. But if salvation isn't part of the package, then I'm not interested. I'll put my trust in God, for he has my eternal interest at heart. If he doesn't heal me physically, then he'll tell me one day why not.

But I believe miracles do happen, and I'd like to encourage you all never to underestimate what God can do. Healing does happen today, and we can all pray for healing. It is God who does the work, not us, so we have no need to be super-righteous or holy, or even to have great faith. We can lay hands on someone if we feel this is the right thing to do. But there is no formula for our words or action. All we need to do is simply to ask God to heal.

You don't need lots of faith to pray for or receive healing. Don't give up if nothing seems to be happening to the people you are praying for. Maybe if you see them again, have enough confidence to ask how they are going. You might not see the results straight-away or ever, but neither do doctors and we still believe doctors can fix us. Doctors can't cure everything, but we don't give up on them. Don't give up on God.

If you don't see healing, don't blame anyone. You didn't have too little faith, the person you were praying for didn't have too little faith either. It just didn't happen maybe the way you expected it. Spiritual and emotional healing might be going on deep down where you can't see it.

For me, I am declining daily, but much slower than expected. All of this is God's work, and my neurologist in Sydney never ceases to be amazed at my level of functioning despite steady brain deterioration. So I do believe miracles happen, and I'd like to encourage you to try not to underestimate God. I am always surprised by how he works in my life, even in the midst of my daily struggles with this disease.

God has given me enough time to help change views about people living with dementia, that they are people worthy of value and dignity. Like Jesus, we need to love them as they are, to see them as real human beings, and to connect with them at the deep level of spirit to spirit.

Frequently Asked Questions

When I give talks, people always ask lots of questions about dementia. Like them, I did not know anything about Alzheimer's or other dementias before the fateful day when the doctor told me I had Alzheimer's Disease and later that I had fronto-temporal dementia.

I have found the national website of Alzheimer's Australia (www.alzheimers.org.au) to be a very helpful source of information. It has drawn from other sources in the UK, Scotland and the USA to compile a very comprehensive amount of information. People with dementia were involved in developing the site, so I find it easy to use, without pictures or moving objects that can distract me. I have used this website, together with my own 'insider's perspective', as a major source to put together the following material to help answer a few of the most frequently asked questions. There are many other sites on the world wide web about dementia.

There is also a very special web site to me, www.dasninternational.org, which was developed by people with dementia, for people with dementia. We are linked together as an email community and chat room throughout the world as part of the Dementia Advocacy and Support Network International. Some of my talks are on this website.

Who gets dementia?

Most people with dementia are older, but it is important to remember that most older people do not get dementia. It is not a normal part of aging.

Dementia can happen to anybody, but it is more common after the age of 65 years. One in four people over the age of 85 have the condition. People in their 30s, 40s and 50s can also have dementia. I was only 46 when I was diagnosed with dementia, and in DASNI I knew a young woman in her early 20s who had dementia.

What is dementia?

Dementia is the 'umbrella' term used for a large group of illnesses, including Alzheimer's Disease, which cause a progressive decline in a person's mental functioning, such as a loss of memory, intellect, rationality, social skills and normal emotional reactions.

There are various types of dementia, but Alzheimer's Disease is the most common type. The effects of the different types of dementia are similar, but not identical, as each one tends to affect different parts of the brain.

What is younger or early-onset dementia?

The term younger or early-onset dementia describes any form of dementia occurring in people under the age of 65.

What is senile dementia?

In the past, senile dementia was regarded as being associated with old age, and pre-senile dementia was a disease with similar symptoms in a younger person.

It is now realised that dementia can occur at any age, and is the result of a number of types of illnesses, such as Alzheimer's Disease, none of which is a normal part of aging. So it is vital to have an accurate diagnosis for any symptoms of dementia, even in elderly people, as treatment is available both to alleviate symptoms and, in some cases, to prevent further damage. For example, if the dementia is the result of poor nutrition in an elderly person, this can be readily addressed.

What is early-stage dementia?

The term early-stage dementia describes any form of dementia in its earlier stages, when the person can still do most things for themselves.

Is dementia the same as Alzheimer's Disease?

Dementia is the word used to describe the types of illnesses that cause brain damage leading to symptoms of memory loss, confusion, language problems and behavioural change. There are about 70 different causes or types of dementia. Alzheimer's Disease is the most common form of dementia, and one specific type of dementia.

Can dementia be inherited?

It depends on the type of dementia.

For example, although about a third of people with Alzheimer's Disease have a close relative with dementia, the inherited type of Alzheimer's Disease is very rare. Alzheimer's Disease occurs relatively frequently in elderly people, regardless of family history.

About 20–50 per cent of people with fronto-temporal dementia have a family history of the disease.

In some rare cases of younger onset Alzheimer's Disease there is a clear pattern of each child having a 50 per cent chance of inheriting the disorder. For those at risk, genetic testing and counselling is available.

What is Alzheimer's Disease?

Alzheimer's Disease is the most common type of dementia, accounting for 50–70 per cent of all cases. It is a physical, progressive, degenerative disease, which affects the brain, resulting in impaired memory, thinking and behaviour. Alois Alzheimer first described it in 1907, in a 56-year-old woman.

As brain cells die, the substance of the brain shrinks. Abnormal material builds up as tangles form in the centre of the brain cells and plaques accumulate outside the brain cells, disrupting messages within the brain and damaging connections between brain cells. Chemical changes also occur in the brain. This leads to the eventual death of the brain cells.

Memory of recent events is the first to be affected, but as the disease progresses, long-term memory is also lost. The disease also affects many of the brain's other functions and consequently many other aspects of the person's functioning are disturbed.

Alzheimer's Disease usually occurs after age 65, and affects people who may or may not have a family history of the disease. A very rare form of Alzheimer's Disease is genetic, and if a parent has a mutated gene, each child has a 50 per cent chance of eventually developing the disease, usually in their 40s or 50s.

In the early stages the symptoms of Alzheimer's Disease can be very subtle, and similar to other types of dementia. However, it often begins with persistent and frequent memory difficulties, especially of recent events, and difficulty in finding the right words for everyday objects.

Symptoms that can also be found in other types of dementia may include vagueness and losing the point of everyday conversation (my speed of processing what you say is slower); apparent loss of enthusiasm for previously enjoyed activities (often called apathy – everyday life takes so much of my energy); taking longer to do routine tasks (nothing is automatic anymore, so everything takes more effort and thought); forgetting well-known people or places (I have lost the 'label', but still know someone or some place is important to me); inability to process questions and instructions (there is not enough space in my brain to hold onto all this information); deterioration of social skills (there is not enough thinking space to remember what to do and say) and emotional unpredictability (I have less control and am more immediate in my reactions).

The disease progresses at a different pace according to the individual and the areas of the brain affected, and abilities may fluctuate from day to day, or even within the one day, becoming worse in times of stress, fatigue or ill-health. I certainly have my good and bad days. However, the disease does lead eventually to complete dependence and finally death, usually from another illness such as pneumonia. A person may live from 3 to 20 years with Alzheimer's Disease, with the average being 7 to 10 years. However, such estimates depend on exactly when during the course of the disease the person was diagnosed.

Scientists are rapidly learning more about the chemical changes which damage brain cells in Alzheimer's Disease but apart from the few individuals with genetic Alzheimer's Disease, it is not known why one individual gets Alzheimer's Disease late in life and another does not. A variety of suspected causes are being investigated including factors in the environment, biochemical disturbances and immune processes. The cause may vary from person to person and may be due to one factor or a number of factors.

What is vascular dementia?

Vascular dementia is the second most common form of dementia. It is due to problems in the circulation of blood to the brain causing a deterioration of mental abilities as a result of multiple strokes, or infarcts, in the brain. A stroke refers to the death of a piece of brain tissue supplied by a blood vessel or blood vessels where the blood supply is blocked or interrupted. These strokes may cause damage to specific areas of the brain responsible for speech or language as well as producing generalised symptoms of dementia.

Vascular dementia may appear similar to Alzheimer's Disease. A mixture of Alzheimer's Disease and vascular dementia is a common cause of dementia, and it can sometimes be difficult to separate the two. 'Internet' friends of mine have this diagnosis, and have very similar problems to those of us with other types of dementia.

Probably the most common form of vascular dementia is multi-infarct dementia caused by a number of small strokes, called mini-strokes or transient ischaemic attacks, which cause damage to the cortex of the brain – the area associated with learning, memory and language. Symptoms may include severe depression, mood swings and epilepsy.

Another type is Binswanger's disease (or sub cortical vascular dementia), which may be relatively common. It is associated with stroke-related changes, affecting the 'white matter' deep within the brain, and is caused by high blood pressure, thickening of the arteries and inadequate blood flow. Symptoms often include: slowness and lethargy; difficulty walking; emotional ups and downs; lack of bladder control early in the course of the disease; gradually progressive dementia developing later.

Several factors increase the risk for vascular dementia, including: high blood pressure, smoking, diabetes mellitus, high cholesterol, history of mild warning strokes, evidence of disease in arteries elsewhere, and heart rhythm abnormalities.

Vascular dementia usually progresses gradually in a step-wise fashion in which a person's abilities deteriorate after a stroke and then stabilise until the next stroke. Sometimes the steps are so small that the decline appears gradual. On average though, people with vascular dementia decline more rapidly than people with Alzheimer's Disease, often dying from a heart attack or major stroke.

What is dementia with Lewy bodies?

A significant number of people diagnosed with dementia are found to have tiny spherical structures called Lewy bodies in the nerve cells of their brains. It is thought these may contribute to the death of brain cells. They are named after the doctor who first wrote about them. It is sometimes referred to as diffuse Lewy body disease.

Dementia with Lewy bodies sometimes co-occurs with Alzheimer's Disease and vascular dementia. The symptoms of dementia with Lewy bodies include: fluctuations in the condition; difficulties with concentration and attention; extreme confusion; difficulties judging distances, often resulting in falls; visual hallucinations; delusions; depression, and tremors and stiffness similar to that seen in Parkinson's Disease.

Dementia with Lewy bodies is often mild at the outset and can be extremely variable from day to day. Friends of mine with this type of dementia have been diagnosed on the basis of symptoms such as hallucinations, delusions and tremors occurring relatively early on in the disease. The disease is progressive, eventually leading to complete dependence. Death is usually as a result of another illness such as pneumonia or an infection. The average lifespan after the onset of symptoms is about seven years. At present there is no known cause of dementia with Lewy bodies and no risk factors have been identified.

What is fronto-temporal dementia?

Fronto-temporal dementia is due to a progressive degeneration of the temporal and frontal lobes of the brain. Damage to the temporal lobe affects language and emotion, and damage to the frontal lobe leads to alterations in behaviour and loss of judgement. It usually begins between 40 and 65 years of age. I was 46 when diagnosed (initially it was thought to be Alzheimer's Disease).

An early symptom is behavioural change, including impulsivity, hyperactivity and being obsessive. I am no longer a 'can do' person, and also find it very hard to restrain my impulses, in terms of, say, picking wool off a stranger's coat, stepping in people's way or speaking loudly. I am at times manic, focused, agitated and active, and have this obsession about going to collect our mail.

Language problems often occur early in the disease. Instead of being able to find the right word to describe an object, I often have to describe it instead. I once rated very highly in terms of verbal fluency, but now have great difficulty – the picture for something is in my head, but the word for it has gone. Mutism usually develops, and I am dreading this, as I think I will be very frustrated at not being able to communicate my feelings. However, apparently the person at this stage may still be able to retain some understanding of what is spoken to them.

There is increasing impairment in 'executive functions', such as distractibility (I am easily distracted by what is going on around me); inflexibility (often I cannot cope with alternative views to my own); or difficulty adapting to changing circumstances (I need my routines). Planning and problem solving ability decreases (I cannot work, and rely on my husband for cooking, driving, washing, and other such complex activities).

Fronto-temporal dementia includes frontal lobe dementia, Pick's Disease, cortico-basal degeneration, progressive aphasia, and semantic dementia. It may also be associated with motor neurone disease or amyotrophic lateral sclerosis (Lou Gehrig's Disease).

The course of these dementias is an inevitable progressive deterioration. From the onset of the disease, life expectancy can be 2 to 15 years, with an average of 6 to 12 years. Death usually comes from another illness such as an infection.

It is caused by abnormalities in the tau protein.

What is alcohol-related dementia?

Alcohol-related dementia is related to the excessive drinking of alcohol, particularly if associated with a diet deficient in thiamine (Vitamin B1). It is currently unclear as to whether alcohol has a direct toxic effect on the brain cells or whether the damage is due to lack of thiamine, vitamin B1. The symptoms can vary from person to person but generally will include: impaired ability to learn new things; personality changes; problems with memory; difficulty with tasks which require planning, organising, judgement and social skills; problems with balance, and decreased initiative and spontaneity.

Males who drink more than six standard alcoholic drinks a day, and women who drink more than four alcoholic drinks a day seem to be at increased risk. If drinking stops, there may be some improvement. Taking thiamine appears to help prevent and improve the condition.

What is AIDS-related dementia?

When someone has acquired immune deficiency syndrome (AIDS) they may develop a complication to the disease which is known as AIDS-related dementia. Symptoms include: difficulty concentrating and remembering; slowed thinking and task completion; difficulty keeping track of daily activities; irritability; difficulty with balance; poor coordination and a change in handwriting, and depression.

Down's Syndrome-related Alzheimer's Disease?

Studies show that by the age of 40, most people with Down's Syndrome have the changes in the brain associated with Alzheimer's Disease. They have an extra copy of chromosome 21, so make much more amyloid precursor protein, and this seems to result in an excess of abnormal amyloid break-down product, which appears to cause earlier appearance of the brain changes typical of Alzheimer's Disease. However, a significant number of people with Down's Syndrome are older than 40 and show no signs of having Alzheimer's Disease. It is not currently understood why changes to the brain that are typical of Alzheimer's Disease do not necessarily produce the disease in people with Down's Syndrome.

What are the early signs of dementia?

The early signs of dementia are subtle, vary a great deal and may not be immediately obvious. They include problems with memory, confusion, personality change, apathy and withdrawal, and loss of ability to do everyday tasks. Sometimes people fail to recognise that these symptoms indicate that something is wrong, and mistakenly assume that these are a normal part of the aging process. Families often say the person has 'changed' and 'is different', but cannot point to anything major, just an accumulation of small changes.

- One of the main symptoms of dementia is memory loss. We all forget things from time to time, but the loss of memory with dementia is persistent and progressive, not just occasional. It's normal to occasionally forget appointments or a friend's phone number and remember them later, but a person with dementia may forget things more often and not remember them at all. There is simply a blank, a 'black hole' where events, places and names used to be.

- People can get distracted from time to time and they may forget to serve part of a meal. A person with dementia may have trouble with all steps involved in preparing a meal. I need to be very focused to do such a complex task and any distraction means it is forgotten.

- It's normal to forget the day of the week – for a moment. But a person with dementia may have difficulty finding their way to a familiar place, or feel confused about where they are. I never can work out what day or time it is, and can feel very confused if left alone even in a familiar place.

- Everyone has trouble finding the right word sometimes, but a person with dementia may forget simple words or substitute inappropriate words, making sentences difficult to understand. Mine are scrambled grammatically and with the totally wrong words.

- Balancing a cheque-book can be difficult for anyone, but a person with dementia may have trouble knowing what the numbers mean and what needs to be done with them. I try very hard, but sometimes numbers are just sounds or squiggles, and I cannot calculate any more.

- Dementia affects a person's memory and concentration and this in turn affects their judgement. Many activities, such as driving, require good judgement and when this ability is affected, the person will be a risk, not only to themselves, but to others on the road. I find driving to be a very complex skill that requires concentration and an ability to react quickly, which I can no longer do.

- Anyone can temporarily misplace a wallet or keys. A person with dementia may put things in inappropriate places. I put something down, when distracted by another task, then forget where I put it, and it turns up in the most peculiar place!

- Everyone becomes sad or moody from time to time. Someone with dementia can exhibit rapid mood swings for no apparent reason. They can become confused, suspicious or withdrawn. My emotions just seem very scrambled and mixed up.

- People's personalities can change a little with age, but with dementia a person may become suspicious or fearful, apathetic and uncommunicative, or dis-inhibited, over-familiar and more outgoing. I have changed a great deal, from being very much in control and task-oriented, to a person who is dependent and more led by impulse and emotion.

- It's normal to tire of some activities, but dementia may cause a person to lose interest in previously enjoyed activities. Everything takes so much effort, that even daily life is a chore.

How is dementia diagnosed?

Many treatable conditions have symptoms similar to dementia, so it is important to consult a doctor to obtain a diagnosis at an early stage. There is currently no single test to identify Alzheimer's Disease or any other dementia. The diagnosis is made only after careful clinical consultation and an assessment which might include the following:

- A detailed medical history, provided if possible by the person with the symptoms and a close relative or friend. This helps to establish whether there is a slow or sudden onset of symptoms and their progression. I went with my daughter, who was able to verify my increasing difficulties.

- A thorough physical and neurological examination, including tests of the senses and movements to rule out other causes of dementia and to identify medical illnesses which may worsen the confusion associated with dementia. I have had regular testing each year.

- Laboratory tests including a variety of blood and urine tests called a 'dementia screen' to test for a variety of possible illnesses which could be responsible for the symptoms. I had a range of such tests, including for AIDS.

- Neuropsychological testing to identify retained abilities and specific problem areas such as comprehension, insight and judgement. These psychometric tests were critical in finding out which areas of my brain were most affected.

- Other specialised tests such as a chest x-ray, ECG, or CT scan. These have shown progressive damage over the years. This is not always the case. Sometimes there are symptoms but little damage to the brain.

- A mental status test to check the range of intellectual functions affected by the dementia such as memory, the ability to read, write and calculate. This simple test was not very helpful in diagnosing me, because of my previous ability. The psychometric tests were of more value.

- Psychiatric assessment to identify treatable disorders which can mimic dementia, such as depression, and also to manage psychiatric symptoms such as anxiety or delusions, which may occur alongside a dementing illness. It is really important to rule out depression which can cause 'pseudo-dementia'.

A definite diagnosis of the actual type of dementia can only be made by examining the brain, after death. However, the type and course of the symptoms may assist in determining the probable diagnosis. The above assessments will help to eliminate other conditions with similar symptoms such as nutritional deficiencies or depression.

After eliminating other causes, a clinical diagnosis of Alzheimer's Disease can be made with about 80–90 per cent accuracy. Sometimes vascular dementia is difficult to distinguish from Alzheimer's Disease, and it is quite possible for a person to have both vascular dementia and Alzheimer's Disease. Lewy Body dementia is also very similar to Alzheimer's Disease and it has sometimes been difficult in the past to distinguish the two. Fronto-temporal dementia again can be hard to differentiate and I was initially diagnosed with Alzheimer's Disease, then fronto-temporal dementia, but the latter usually begins at an earlier age and is primarily a disease of behaviour and language dysfunction, rather than memory. For other dementias, certain laboratory tests, including an examination of cerebrospinal fluid, may be useful, such as in identifying AIDS-related dementia.

How can I get the person to see the doctor?

Some people may be resistant to the idea of visiting a doctor. In some cases, people do not realise, or else deny, there is anything wrong with them. This can be due to the brain changes of dementia that interfere with the ability to recognise or appreciate one's memory problems. Others, with retained insight, may be afraid of having their fears confirmed.

One of the most effective ways to overcome this problem is to find a physical reason for a visit to the doctor, such as a general health check, or a review of long-term medication. Another way is to suggest that it is time for you *both* to have a physical check up. A calm, caring attitude at this time can help overcome very real worries and fears. You may need to talk to the doctor about your concerns before this check-up, so that the doctor can be prepared, and able to gently explore the key issues.

Should I tell the person with dementia about the diagnosis?

There are some good reasons to tell the person with dementia about the diagnosis. Many people are already aware that something is wrong. The diagnosis of dementia can come as a relief as they now know what is causing the problem. Access to information, support and new treatments are helped when the person knows about their condition.

Early intervention can enhance quality of life, and knowing about the condition can allow for planning for the future, and for an honest and open discussion of the experience of dementia between family and friends.

As a person with dementia, I think it is patronising not to tell us, and that it is a matter of human rights to allow us to know what is wrong with us in time to make choices about treatment and management of our condition. But I know some carers don't agree, because they feel that it might cause us extra distress and unnecessary trauma, when we are already struggling, knowing something is not right 'in our head'. The important issue is to do what you think the person with dementia would want you to do, think about their character before they became sick, and whether they would want to know, and whether diagnosis, treatment and support, knowing they are not alone, would help them.

Is there a cure or treatment for dementia?

At present there is no cure for most forms of dementia, but there is treatment.

With vascular dementia, treatment to prevent additional strokes is very important. Medicines to control high blood pressure, high cholesterol, heart disease and diabetes can be prescribed. A healthy diet, exercise and avoidance of smoking and excessive alcohol also lessen the risk of further strokes. Sometimes aspirin or other drugs are prescribed to prevent clots from forming in the small blood vessels.

The cholinergic drugs, or acetyl cholinesterase inhibitors, have a modest but definite effect on the core symptoms of mild to moderate dementia, for many people I know. Currently available cholinesterase inhibitors are: donepezil (Aricept, which I take each day), rivastigmine (Exelon), and galantamine (Reminyl). The chemical acetyl choline is a neurotransmitter which is important in transmitting messages between some brain cells, particularly in the areas of the brain vital to memory function and acquiring new information. Autopsy studies have shown that this chemical is deficient in the brains of people with Alzheimer's Disease. The cholinesterase inhibitors prevent its breakdown, and so increase the depleted supplies. These drugs have side effects, including nausea and diarrhoea affecting around 10 per cent of people. I carry loperamide hydrochloride (Imodium) with me everywhere for this reason – others might like to talk to their doctor about this too.

Ebixa (memantine) is another class of drug, which according to the Alzheimer's Australia web site may slow down the progression of symptoms in the middle and later stages of Alzheimer's Disease, and may also help in the mild stages. I find it helps me, although I have fronto-temporal dementia, so perhaps it is also helpful for other dementias as well. Check with your specialist. It works differently from acetyl cholinesterase inhibitors, and taking them both (which I do) may be more effective than an acetyl cholinesterase inhibitor alone. Memantine targets glutamate, which is a neurotransmitter that is present in excessive levels in Alzheimer's Disease. This excess glutamate sticks to the nerve cell neuro-receptors, allowing calcium to move into the brain cells and cause damage. Memantine sticks to the same neuro-receptors, blocking the glutamate and preventing such damage.

The areas in which people may find improvement are in functioning in daily activities (I am able to shower myself now), and an overall change in function (my mind is clearer). A small number of people have experienced side effects, which are usually mild to moderate. These side effects can include hallucinations, confusion, dizziness, headache and tiredness.

There is a lot of research underway investigating what may assist in preventing the onset of Alzheimer's Disease or vascular dementia, or, after diagnosis, may assist in delaying further progression. Because new studies are being published all the time, it is best to use websites to check on the latest information available. Topics to look out for include: Vitamin E, folic acid and Vitamin B12 and gingko biloba. In any event, because of side effects and drug interactions, people are strongly advised to consult their doctor if considering using any other drug/products.

What treatment helps with the other symptoms of dementia?

Dementia often causes a number of behavioural and psychological symptoms, including depression, anxiety, sleeplessness, hallucinations, agitation and aggressive behaviour. Often these symptoms will not require medication and may respond to reassurance, a change in the environment or removal of some distressing stimulus such as pain.

Symptoms of depression are extremely common in dementia. Depression can be effectively treated with anti-depressants, but care must be taken to ensure that this is done with a minimum of side effects. I take moclobemide (Aurorix) as a mood stabiliser.

Anxiety states, accompanied by panic attacks and unreasonable fearfulness can be very distressing and may be helped by a group of drugs known as benzodiazepines. I find that oxazepam (Alepam) helpful in settling me down when I get anxious and stressed by the early evening.

Persistent waking at night and night-time wandering can cause a lot of difficulties. Increased stimulation during the day can help, as people may become dependent on medication and withdrawal may be followed by rebound sleeplessness and anxiety. I rely on temazepam (Temaze) now to switch off my brain at night.

Major tranquillisers, also known as neuroleptics or anti-psychotics, are used to control agitation, aggression, delusions and hallucinations. Commonly used drugs are thioridazine (Melleril) and haliperidol (Serenace). These drugs tend to cause symptoms similar to Parkinson's Disease such as stiffness, shuffling gait and shakiness in higher doses and older people are very prone to these side effects. Newer tranquillisers such as olanzapine (Zyprexa) and risperidone (Risperdal) have fewer side effects and probably work just as well for the relief of symptoms. It is vital that families and doctors work together when considering medications and side effects and other risks are fully discussed.

Should the person with dementia continue to drive?

A diagnosis of dementia does not necessarily mean a person must stop driving immediately. It is important to remember that any decision that results in a person's loss of licence should be made solely for the driver's safety and the safety of others. Driving can be a very difficult practical and emotional issue for people diagnosed with dementia and their families.

Dementia affects driving ability in a number of ways:

- finding the way, even in familiar areas
- remembering which way to turn, and distinguishing left and right
- responding to the unfamiliar
- judging distance from other cars and objects
- judging speed of other cars, and driving slowly
- reaction time, and making slower decisions at traffic lights, intersections or changing lanes

- hand-eye coordination, using the accelerator and brake
- reading maps, and interpreting road signs.

Some people will recognise their declining abilities, others may not. Some people decide to voluntarily relinquish their licence, and recognise benefits in having less stress, and enjoying the scenery along the way. I have stopped driving, except in emergencies. Others may be very reluctant to give up this aspect of their independence. Legal implications need to be checked with local authorities and/or the local Alzheimer's association.

Can a person with dementia plan ahead?

With an early diagnosis, the person with dementia should be able to participate in the planning and make sure that their wishes are carried out. This can make it easier for families and carers to manage the affairs of the person with dementia later on. Wherever possible, seek advice very early on, while the person with dementia can still participate in the discussion and is legally competent to sign any documents.

Dementia affects people differently. One person may begin to lose the ability to handle money matters or make competent business decisions at an early stage, another may keep these skills much longer. However, sooner or later, the abilities of the person with dementia will decline and they may be unable to make their own decisions about their financial, legal and medical matters.

It is useful to set up a legal arrangement such as an enduring power of attorney. One of the benefits of the enduring power of attorney is that it allows the person with dementia to choose, ahead of time, someone to act on their behalf when they are no longer able to do so themselves. I set one up for my eldest daughter in the first year after diagnosis, and then set up another one when I married Paul. There are different documents to cover legal, financial and medical issues.

Where To Go For Help

For more information on any issues relating to dementia I encourage you to make contact with your national Alzheimer's Association. Their address may be in your telephone directory, or you can pick up an internet link through Alzheimer's Disease International at www.alz.co.uk.

Endnotes

1   C. Boden, 1998, *Who will I be when I die?*, HarperCollins, East Melbourne, Victoria.

2   L. Jackson, March 2001, private email correspondence.

3   Y. Kawamura, October 2003, private email correspondence.

4   R. Reagan, 1994, Letter from President Ronald Reagan to the American people, reproduced in *Alzheimer's Disease, The brain killer*, in C.J. Vas, S. Rajkumar, P. Tanyakitpisal and V. Chandra, (eds) World Health Organization, SEA/Ment/116, 2001.

5   C. Boden, 1998, *op. cit.*, p.100.

6   C. Boden, 1998, *op. cit.*, p.117.

7   C. Boden, 1998, *op. cit.*, p.34.

8   S. Hughes, 1998, *Every day with Jesus*, May/June, Crusade for World Revival (CWR), Surrey.

9   C. Boden, 1998, *op. cit.*, p.10.

10 Alzheimer's Australia, 2001, 'Consumer focus report,' www.alzheimers.org.au.

11 C. Mulliken, January 2001, private email correspondence.

12 M.L. King, 1994, *Letter from the Birmingham Jail*, San Francisco, HarperSanFrancisco.

13 M. Friedell and C. Bryden, 2001, Talk to Australian National Conference, April 2001, www.dasninternational.org.

14 T. Bowden, 2001, Australian Broadcasting Corporation (ABC) 7.30 Report, 'Positive attitude to living with dementia,' 11 June, www.abc.net.au/7.30/S311227.htm.

15 DASNI, 23 June 2001, Proposal to ADI, private correspondence.

16 P. Hardt, July 2001, private email correspondence.

17 In S. Ratcliffe (ed.), 2000, *The Oxford dictionary of thematic quotations*, Oxford University Press, Oxford, p.86.

18 In S. Stewart, 2003, *Words to the wise, A collection of African proverbs*, Spearhead, Claremont, p.72.

19 B. McNaughton, November 2001, private email correspondence.

20 W. Fleming and V. Schofield, October 2001, private email correspondence.

21 V. Schofield, March 2003, private email correspondence.

22 V. Schofield, June 2004, private email correspondence.

23 N. Mandela, 1994, State of the Nation Address, Cape Town, 24 May, www.anc.org.za.

24 L. Smith, January 2001, private email correspondence in response to request from C. Jonas-Simpson, Early onset Alzheimer's Disease, http://www.swchsc.on.ca/research/eoad.html.

25 M. Lockhart, August 2000, private email correspondence.

26 D. Bagnall, 2004, *The Bulletin*, 22 June, ACP Publishing, Sydney.

27 L. Jackson, August 2000, private email correspondence.

28 John, August 2000, private email correspondence.

29 J. Phillips, August 2000, private email correspondence.

30 M. Friedell, August 2000, private email correspondence.

31 C. Bryden, August 2000, private email correspondence.

32 In S. Stewart, 2003, *op. cit.*, p.46.

33 S. Sabat, 2003, 'Some potential benefits of creating research partnerships with people with Alzheimer's Disease,' *Research Policy and Planning 21*, 2, pp.5–12.

34 C. Bryden, 2002, 'A person-centred approach to counselling, psychotherapy and rehabilitation of people diagnosed with dementia in the early stages,' *Dementia: The International Journal of Social Research and Practice 1*, 2, pp.141–156.

35 M. Friedell, January 2001, private email correspondence.

36 M. Friedell, 'A nine-step rehabilitation program for early Alzheimer's Disease,' http://members.aol.com/MorrisFF/Eight.html.

37 M. Friedell, August 2000, private email correspondence.

38 F. Drysdale, 2001, 'Numero,' http://www.fdc.com.au/numero.

39 M. Goldsmith, 1996, *Hearing the voice of people with dementia*, Jessica Kingsley Publishers, London, pp.58–59.

40 D. Bagnall, 2004, *op. cit.*

41 J.R. Dudley, 1997, *Confronting the stigma in their lives*, Thomas Books, Illinois, p.9.

42 T. Kitwood, 1995, 'A dialectical framework for dementia,' In R.T. Woods *et al.* (eds), *Handbook of clinical psychology of ageing*,' pp.267–282.

43 V. Frankl, 1984, *Man's search for meaning*, Washington Square Press, New York, p.38.

44 E.B. MacKinlay, 2001, *The spiritual dimension of ageing*, Jessica Kingsley Publishers, London.

45 E.B. MacKinlay (ed.), 2002, *Mental health and spirituality in later life*, Haworth Pastoral Press, New York.

46 C. Boden, 1998, p.49. *op. cit.*

47 E.B. MacKinlay (ed.), 2002, *op. cit.*

48 In S. Ratcliffe, 2000, *op. cit.*, p.201.

49 In S. Ratcliffe, 2000, *op. cit.*, p.342.

50 P. Tillich, 1963, *Systemic theology vol.3. op. cit.*, University of Chicago Press, Chicago.

51 M. Friedell, October 2000, private email correspondence.

52 S. Garnett, June 2004, private email correspondence.

53   S. Garnett, July 2004, private email correspondence.

54   In S. Stewart, 2003, *op. cit.*, p.59.

55   V. Frankl, 1984, *op. cit.*

56   V. Frankl, 1984, *op. cit.*, p.87.

57   B. McNaughton, June 2004, private email correspondence.